Prostate Cancer
Thriving Through Treatment to Recovery

Lisa A. Price, ND

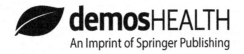

demosHEALTH
An Imprint of Springer Publishing

Visit our website at www.springerpub.com

Demos Health is an imprint of Springer Publishing Company, LLC.

ISBN: 9780826148551
ebook ISBN: 9780826148568

Acquisitions Editor: Beth Barry
Compositor: diacriTech

Medical information provided by Demos Health, in the absence of a visit with a health care professional, must be considered as an educational service only. This book is not designed to replace a physician's independent judgment about the appropriateness or risks of a procedure or therapy for a given patient. Our purpose is to provide you with information that will help you make your own health care decisions.

The information and opinions provided here are believed to be accurate and sound, based on the best judgment available to the authors, editors, and publisher, but readers who fail to consult appropriate health authorities assume the risk of injuries. The publisher is not responsible for errors or omissions. The editors and publisher welcome any reader to report to the publisher any discrepancies or inaccuracies noticed.

Library of Congress Cataloging-in-Publication Data
Names: Price, Lisa A., author.
Title: Prostate cancer : thriving through treatment to recovery / Lisa A. Price, ND.
Description: New York : Demos Health, [2019] | Includes bibliographical
    references and index.
Identifiers: LCCN 2018058247 | ISBN 9780826148551 (alk. paper) |
    ISBN 9780826148568 (ebook)
Subjects: LCSH: Prostate—Cancer—Treatment.
Classification: LCC RC280.P7 P637 2019 | DDC 616.99/463—dc23
LC record available at https://lccn.loc.gov/2018058247

Contact us to receive discount rates on bulk purchases.
We can also customize our books to meet your needs.
For more information please contact: sales@springerpub.com

Publisher's Note: **New and used products purchased from third-party sellers are not guaranteed for quality, authenticity, or access to any included digital components.**

Printed in the United States of America.
18 19 20 21 22 / 5 4 3 2 1

CONTENTS

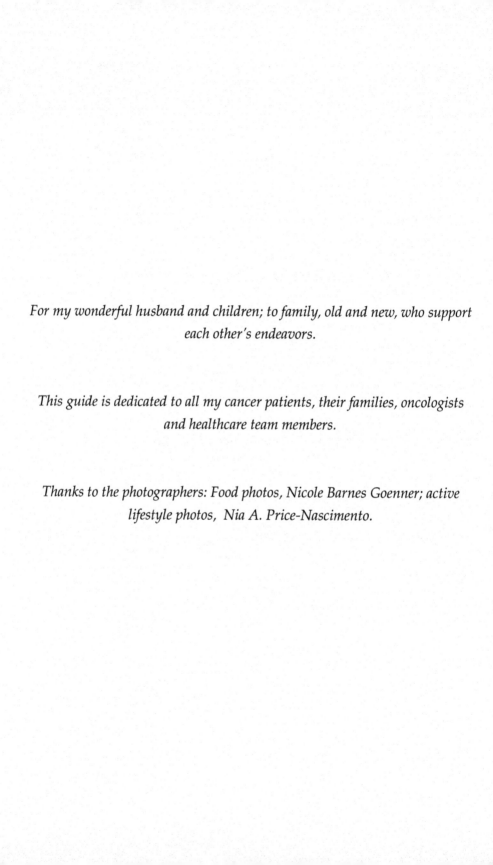

For my wonderful husband and children; to family, old and new, who support each other's endeavors.

This guide is dedicated to all my cancer patients, their families, oncologists and healthcare team members.

Thanks to the photographers: Food photos, Nicole Barnes Goenner; active lifestyle photos, Nia A. Price-Nascimento.

PREFACE

If truth be told, there is no one magic bullet when it comes to perfect health, treatment, or cures. This is particularly pertinent regarding cancer treatment. While conventional therapies are vital, they result in side effects that can greatly affect quality of life and self-identity, and impact recovery and remission. Patients are often told that diet, exercise, and other activities won't make a difference in the development or intensity of these symptoms. Nothing could be further from the truth, and peer-reviewed research supports this. It is therefore of utmost importance that all patients use safe and comprehensive planning during cancer treatment through recovery for best outcomes.

That is where this companion guide comes into play. This book is a culmination of my observations of best therapies as a clinician and as a research scientist in complementary and integrative cancer care. I am motivated to share them with you because a holistic approach makes such a positive difference in the lives of patients undergoing cancer treatment through recovery. Besides my own observations, many scientific studies support the effects of specific culinary nutrition, exercise, and mind-body therapies for patients undergoing treatment for prostate cancer.

This book will help you understand the various treatments for prostate cancer and how they work. I also review the effects of treatment on your immune system and your nutritional status. A diagnosis of cancer often comes with a predictable amount of trauma that can lead to some emotional distress, and I address issues that may result and actions to help mitigate.

Overall, the book moves from explanations of what is happening to solutions. These are divided into three sections: cookbook (nutrition), exercise, and mind body therapy, each tailored specifically to benefits for prostate cancer patients.

It is my hope that patients engage in a holistic plan that they can incorporate for their lifetime. I highly recommend that you find a qualified and licensed provider to help guide you. If you are having trouble finding a healthcare provider in complementary cancer care with expertise in culinary nutrition, please feel free to contact me at www. drlisapricend.com for an online consult.

May you all be on your path to healing and wellness with hope and strength.

ACKNOWLEDGEMENTS

I would like to thank my parents for catalyzing a deep desire for knowledge, encouraging my curiosity, and for being wonderful examples. Glen, Nia, and Cypress, thank you for understanding my need for time. Finally, to my conventional and naturopathic colleagues, thank you for your endless dedication in supporting all our patients. Thank you, Nicole and Nia, for stepping up to the plate.

Introduction

Never believe that a few caring people can't change the world. For, indeed, that's all who ever have.

—*Margaret Mead*

Several years ago, a stage IV prostate cancer patient, who I will call Stan, came to me for complementary care. I have been fortunate to work in cancer centers that are progressive and honor the importance of safe alternative therapies in conjunction with conventional medicine. Stan was receiving the best treatment from the best oncology team, and even went out of state to another prestigious cancer treatment facility for a second opinion. The first and second opinions matched. Both facility's oncologists noted that statistics for his diagnosis were not favorable for long-term survival; therefore, it was highly unlikely his cancer would ever reach the much desired "NED" (No Evidence of Disease) status. Stan and his wife were not deterred. They persisted, following the prescribed conventional treatment plan as well as complying with the complementary plan I supplied. My plan included safe supplementation, dietary support, behavioral modifications, mind–body therapies, and exercise. Stan, I should mention, is also deeply spiritual and insatiably curious, as is his wife.

As the weeks and months progressed, Stan kept to the treatment protocols, and made it through therapy with very few side effects. In and of itself, having only a small amount of side effects during treatment was an enormous achievement.

The time for him to be scanned came, and the results showed NED. He was elated, and his oncology team was baffled. Statistically, this was not supposed to happen. Because this was not "normal," his case was sent to several tumor boards to determine what to do next. As a result, Stan was assessed frequently in the initial months and succeeding months after another scan, and he retained his NED status.

Knowing that my patients are my greatest teachers, I asked Stan what he thought made the difference. His response: "I don't think it was just one thing or one mode of treatment. I think it was a thousand points of light that coalesced to create healing."

His words had a profound and influential impact on me. They concisely articulated my observations in hundreds of patients since practicing for over a decade in conventional settings: All of these therapies matter to the health, well-being, and outcomes of our patients.

Like Stan, there are many patients who receive an unlikely NED diagnosis, as well as patients living long-term with cancer. In fact, in the last several years, the rate of remission and stabilization has increased so significantly that a newly recognized phase of treatment has been added called "survivorship." This is particularly important and relevant in prostate cancer because, in many cases, the cancer is slow growing and a watch-and-wait approach is the option oncologists recommend.

The survivorship trend was noted by a large and important body of professionals in the cancer world called the Commission on Cancer, a credentialing body composed of surgeons. In 2005, understanding the importance of holistic plans to maintain health, which were based on peer-reviewed scientific studies, the Commission suggested that all accredited cancer institutes create what is known as survivorship programs. These programs provide cancer patients with:

- Concise assessment plans with the oncology care team
- Physical need assessments and services (exercise and physical therapy)
- Nutritional analysis and plans
- Emotional well-being services (mind–body therapies)

Many cancer centers have these services, and you should ask your oncologist or healthcare provider about the survivorship programs they are associated with.

Cancer treatment and diagnosis are physically and emotionally traumatic, causing challenges to mental and physical health, and to nutritional status. Conventional treatment, which includes surgery, radiation, chemotherapy, and hormone therapy, is effective in treating cancer. However, treatment can and often results in short- and long-term side effects that can affect quality of life and increase the potential risk of long-term ailments including second cancers. Most of the effects are caused by the treatment's direct tissue necrosis or damage, depression of the immune system, and/or nutrient deficiencies.

It is necessary to address these changes for optimal health to be achieved. We do know that cancer treatment depletes certain important nutrients. Studies by the National Cancer Institute have found that nutrition and, in particular, specific foods, can affect outcome and even help or hurt short- and long-term side effects. Patients receiving nutritional counseling before, during, and after cancer treatment have better outcomes, quality of life, and experience significantly fewer side effects. Furthermore, certain nutrients control the onset of specific side effects from treatment. There are several good studies that validate the importance of nutrition in prevention and remission. One such study, a 2013 survey, demonstrated the need of cancer patients and survivors regarding diet, exercise, and weight management. James–Martin and his team found that patients thought there was a lack of information regarding diet and exercise during and after conventional treatment. As mentioned, those receiving nutritional counseling during and after treatment had better outcomes and reduced side effects. Other holistic interventions also play a significant role in cancer treatment outcomes and the prevention of cancer progression

We know research from the National Cancer Institute and from the European Prospective Investigation into Cancer (EPIC) study demonstrates that exercise is the number one factor correlated with remission and cancer prevention. Exercise, both aerobic and resistance training, is important for preventing and decreasing side effects associated with prostate cancer treatment like muscle wasting, decreased sexual function, and lowered self-esteem. Physical activity can directly affect tumor growth by modulating inflammatory responses in the tumor mass microenvironment. This is an extremely important finding as it relates to recurrence and remission. There are other long-term symptoms that can be addressed by exercise as well. Fatigue, muscle loss, circulation, decreased stamina, and bone loss resulting from cancer treatment is associated with loss of muscle mass. Fatigue associated with muscle loss is associated with increased risk of developing osteopenia and osteoporosis associated with androgen deprivation therapy/hormone therapies for prostate cancer.

Another important reason to address nutrition, exercise, and emotional needs is that these therapies help to decrease the *fear* associated with long-term side effects of cancer treatments, namely chemotherapy, radiation, and hormone therapy. Studies and statistics do show that use of these vital therapies come with long-term risks, including the development of second cancers such as leukemia. The fear of developing side effects during treatment and during recovery creates an immense amount of anxiety. Holistic plans can have a positive affect on quality of life and substantially decrease anxiety and worry for cancer patients.

That is why this book is a vital resource for anyone diagnosed with cancer, because like Stan and many of my other patients, I believe that achieving NED, remission, and living a good quality of life with cancer necessitates a "thousand points of light" approach.

There is an obvious need for a comprehensive holistic resource for cancer patients, oncologists, and even pharmaceutical companies that addresses minimizing short- and long-term side effects associated with treatment, and therefore the negative association patients have with treatment. This guide provides solutions rather than just highlighting the problematic and burdensome side effects of treatment.

This book is written for cancer patients and their families who would like to use a comprehensive, complementary approach like Stan did. This approach is based on the general recommendations of the Commission on Cancer and is guided by statistical data gathered by the National Cancer Institute to address healing through cancer treatment and beyond. These recommendations are supported by hundreds of scientific studies.

This book contains holistic information specific for prostate cancer and will:

- Help you understand your treatment
- Help you understand the possible short- and long-term side effects and provide some solutions to preventing or decreasing them

■ Exist as a guide for appropriate and safe levels of nutrition via food to use during each treatment phase into recovery (includes 30 recipes)

■ Provide you with suggestions for appropriate and safe exercise

■ Articulate questions and feelings you might be experiencing throughout treatment and into recovery, as well as options for therapies that help to restore emotional well-being

ORGANIZATION OF THE BOOK

This book is organized into chapters. Chapters 1 and 2 explain conventional treatments for prostate cancer, how they work, and their physiological and emotional side effects. The remaining chapters are dedicated to helpful solutions, including nutrition and recipes, exercise, and mind–body therapies.

Within the first chapter you will find brief descriptions of each treatment type (chemotherapy, radiation, surgery, and hormone therapy) and its effects on your body. The second chapter focuses on the impact a cancer diagnosis has on mental health, and how treatment affects your immune system and emotional well-being.

Chapter 3 contains recipes with information related to treatment, side effects, and nutritional content. Chapter 4 focuses on exercise specifically geared to reducing side effects of treatment and promotion of remission. Each exercise is described and includes benefits and a suggested heart rate or goal frequency.

Finally, because there are unique mental health challenges that arise from diagnosis and treatment, the final chapter is devoted to different mind–body therapies for emotional well-being. Each suggestion includes a description of the therapy, its goal or purpose, and provides information on how to contact appropriate professionals in your area.

The book concludes with helpful appendices to guide you to support organizations and resources for further information.

This book is best used throughout the duration of treatment, though is also very beneficial through recovery and during maintenance as well.

I really never saw myself as a guy who'd ever have to pay attention to what he ate, or someone who'd do any other exercise than going to the gym. When I got diagnosed, I got stopped dead in my tracks and I knew I had to make some changes. I'd say the two biggest things that have helped me during treatment have been changing to a whole food diet and adding yoga. My energy and mood have really stabilized and I started dealing a lot better with the anxiety I had from my diagnosis.

—A. G.

CHAPTER 1

Understanding Chemotherapy, Surgery, Radiation, and Hormone Therapy

Goals allow you to control the direction of change in your favor.

—*Brian Tracey*

Prostate cancer is the most common male cancer, accounting for 24% of all new cancer diagnoses. Prostate cancer treatment, however, does not fall into a one-size-fits-all category. Treatment depends on the extent of and progression of the disease, on the individual, and on other illnesses that the individual might have.

What is for certain is that many men diagnosed with prostate cancer will live for many years or decades with or after being treated for the cancer! Even more promising, biotechnology and immune therapies are moving ahead at the speed of light, enabling treatments to be more effective, less invasive, and more individualized.

Prostate cancer patients fall into several categories based on the location of the disease, extent of the disease, age of the patient, and other illnesses. In general, there are six different types of treatments:

- Observation
- Active surveillance
- Surgery
- Radiation therapy
- Hormone therapy
- Chemotherapy

So how is it determined which treatment is best for you?

Newly diagnosed patients see an oncologist or urologist for comprehensive care and plans. Prostate cancer is monitored by blood tests to measure the level of prostate serum antigen (PSA), along with a digital exam, and sometimes imaging via PET scans or MRIs.

Patients may be diagnosed with localized or locally advanced prostate cancer. Localized, slow-growing cancers will undergo what oncologists term observation. This applies to men with low-risk prostate cancer who have a life expectancy of less than 10 years. Patients are watched and monitored.

Active surveillance is an option for men who have been diagnosed with very a low PSA rate or who have low aggressive prostate cancer. In 50% to 66% of these patients, tumor growth does not progress or warrant treatment. These patients and their oncologists decide not to immediately undergo radical treatment like surgery. They subsequently are monitored frequently using PSA and digital exams, along with a biopsy of the prostate every 1 to 3 years. Side effects of active surveillance are minimal besides those associated with an enlarged prostate such as frequent urination or some erectile dysfunction.

There are several types of treatment options, referred to as localized treatment, that directly target the tumor and surrounding tissue. These include surgery and radiation. Hormone therapy and chemotherapies tend to be more systemic, meaning they affect the whole body.

Surgery is selected as an option when the cancer is not aggressive, is localized, and for younger patients. However, in many cases, surgery is part of the initial effective treatment.

LOCALIZED TREATMENTS

Surgery for this cancer is the removal of part or of the entire prostate (prostatectomy), seminal vesicles, and sometimes the removal of lymph nodes, while attempting to spare nerves, particularly those involved in erectile function that run alongside the prostate. Surgery is usually done robotically, and recovery time is about 1 to 2 days. After a 1- to 2-day hospital stay, patients go home with a catheter to help drain urine for the next 7 to 10 days. Side effects of this treatment can include urine leakage (urinary incontinence) and often require the patient to wear some sort of pad. These symptoms usually improve over several weeks to several months. Patients can receive physical therapy to help speed up resolution of this issue; however most surgeons will recommend against moderate to aggressive physical exercise for the first 2 months. If lymph nodes are involved in the cancer spread, the oncology team will decide if surgery can be teamed with hormone therapy and/or radiation. Erectile dysfunction is another side effect that occurs after surgery if the tumor is large and extends beyond the prostate. In these circumstances, nerve sparing is impossible. Oncologists will use PSA values and scans to assess these patients in the future.

Oncologists and patients may choose to use radiation therapy as opposed to or in conjunction with surgery. Radiation therapy involves killing of cancer cells with ionizing radiation that damages the cancer cells' DNA so that they cannot replicate. Radiation is used for tumors that are localized or that locally advance, and consists of external beam therapy and brachytherapy. External beam therapy involves the application of radiation generated from a machine outside of the body. Brachytherapy involves implanting small radioactive "seeds" or particles into the prostate. Following is a summary of each treatment.

External Beam Radiation

Patients are treated on an outpatient basis during this therapy and healing is quick. Radiation therapy is delivered over 40 to 45 treatments every work day (Monday through Friday). Schedules are modified in consideration of timing, side effects, and other matters.

There are many different types of external beam radiation therapy that might be selected as an option. Some of the options for external beam radiation therapy are:

- Intensity-modulated radiation therapy (IMRT)
- Image-guided radiation therapy (IFRT)
- Stereotactic body radiation therapy(SBRT)
- Proton beam

Side effects of radiation therapy can include increased frequency and urgency of urination or bowel movements during treatment up until around 4 to 6 weeks after treatment is done. Unlike surgery, urinary incontinence is a rare side effect with less than 1% of patients developing it. Radiation therapy can also cause erectile dysfunction. Studies show that erectile dysfunction evolves slowly over time with radiation therapy in men who have good erectile function before treatment. Erectile dysfunction after radiation treatment is estimated to occur in 67% to 85% of patients and may take up to 24 months to develop. Radiation therapy can damage vascular structures leading into and away from the penis.

Brachytherapy

Brachytherapy is a form of radiation treatment that implants small "seeds" of radiation directly into the tumor and surrounding tissue in the prostate. These seeds emit radiation that kill the tumor over the course of several months. The small particles are usually depleted in about a year and the remaining seeds stay in the prostate but are harmless and radioactivity-free by this point. The placement of the seeds is done in one to four sessions.

Erectile dysfunction rates vary from 6% to 51% after brachytherapy. Other side effects resulting from brachytherapy can include increased urinary frequency and obstruction, and sometimes rectal injury.

SYSTEMIC TREATMENTS

Systemic treatments are generally used when oncologists detect a progression in tumor growth and/or PSA levels, when patients decline the surgery treatment option, or when patients have already received other treatment options. Hormone therapy in general works to block production of testosterone and its action on receptors, which help tumor cells to grow. Chemotherapy, the other systemic treatment, damages DNA, preventing the rapid growth of tumor cells. Let us take a closer look at both treatments.

Hormone Therapy

Hormone therapy is perhaps the most commonly used therapy before, during, and after local cancer treatment. The objective of this therapy is not to cure the cancer but to slow down the growth of the tumor and to reduce the tumor size. In some cases, it is a preparation for external beam radiation therapy or brachytherapy. It is important in managing advancing disease (i.e., tumor has spread beyond the prostate). This option is used with patients undergoing radiation or surgery, and with recurrent cancer, or increasing PSA values with no evidence of disease with imaging. It is also known as androgen deprivation therapy and is designed to stop the effect testosterone has on the growth of prostate cancer cells. This treatment is helpful; however, over time the tumor cells learn to grow in a low testosterone environment, and thus the effectiveness of hormone therapy can decrease. If progression continues even with hormone therapy, these patients require more aggressive therapies like chemotherapies, immunotherapy, bone-targeted agents, and investigational drugs/clinical trials.

There are various types of hormone therapy:

- *Orchiectomy*—surgical removal of the testicles. Most men do not select this relatively low-cost therapy because of its permanence and its side effects.

- *Luteinizing hormone releasing hormone (LHRH)*—these work by blocking the luteinizing hormone, which is responsible for sending a signal to the testes to make testosterone. Some examples of these kinds of therapies include Eligard, Lupron, and Zoladex. They are injectables and are usually administered monthly, weekly, biannually or once a year.

- *Antiandrogens*—these work by blocking the action of testosterone in prostate cancer cells. They can be used in combination with LHRH therapies. An example of treatment is bicalutamide.

Hormone therapy causes a significant reduction in serum testosterone that commonly results in reduced sexual desire and sexual function. About 85% of men receiving hormone therapy experience alterations in erectile function. Delayed orgasm or inability to attain orgasm and reduced orgasmic intensity are also common sexual consequences of treatment and may show up after 3 months of treatment. The mechanism causing these changes involves reduction in oxygenation of the penis' smooth muscle cells.

Side effects depend on the type of hormone, but may include hot flashes, loss of bone mass, mood swings, weight gain, gynecomastia, fatigue, muscle loss, and erectile dysfunction.

NONSTANDARD OPTIONS

In my practice, I have been asked frequently about the validity of non-standard therapies in the treatment of prostate cancer. Because of my conventional training as a biochemist, my answer is always the same: Nonstandard options are therapies not supported by rigorous scientific studies and statistics, and therefore involve significant risk, along with lack of guidance when choosing them. These include:

Cryotherapy

Cryotherapy uses extremely cold temperatures to freeze and destroy cancer tissue in the prostate. As mentioned, with almost all nonstandard options, there are not many long-term studies that follow cryotherapy as a treatment for prostate cancer.

High-Intensity-Focused Ultrasound

High-intensity-focused ultrasound is a noninvasive, radiation-free method to destroy prostate tissue and treat prostate disease. The physician uses image guidance to direct a focused beam of ultrasound energy to the area of the prostate gland affected by cancer. While this procedure is Food and Drug Administration (FDA)-approved, it is still controversial among practitioners.

Whatever treatment option is presented, make sure you understand the treatment and its side effects. Most cancer centers work with physical therapists, social workers, and others that can help alleviate or treat side effects and emotional aspects that arise.

Things had been changing between me and my wife since the diagnosis. When I was put on Lupron I had mood changes, felt like my muscles were decreasing. I really felt less masculine, and I began to isolate myself. My self-esteem decreased. With some encouragement I went to see a counselor that had experience with men going through prostate cancer treatment. He helped me to articulate what was happening, and to explore some options to help decrease side effects. We also discussed issues around intimacy and solutions. Things are different, but they are good with my relationship now. I think any man that is going through hormone therapy needs a little help with the changes that happen.

—T. H.

CHAPTER 2

Emotional Aftermath and Effects on the Immune System

Only in the darkness can you see the stars.

—*Martin Luther King, Jr.*

Prostate cancer is not selective. I have had patients who have never paid attention to their diets and get minimal exercise, to patients who are relatively young, athletic, with no other medical issues. Regardless of who you are or your chosen lifestyle, you are most likely to initially experience some degree of shock, helplessness, and anxiety when told you have prostate cancer. Let us face it, most of us do not plan on developing cancer and thus have not researched treatments, side effects, or other important information to gain an understanding of what to expect. At diagnosis, the cancer "learning curve" is steep for the patient. This can create a great deal of anxiety, especially for a person who has been independent up to this point in his life.

One of my patients admitted that he was more nervous about the side effects of treatment than diagnosis. He was most worried about the effect on his relationship and his personal masculine image. He mentioned that he had not found adequate solutions in his research to deal with problems of sexual function and self-esteem. He was relieved to find that therapies do exist, and that their interventions are supported by scientific studies. Though the therapies were ones that he had never thought to incorporate into his life, like counseling and yoga, he was motivated to achieve solutions. In the end, his side effects decreased, he incorporated healthy therapies that addressed a broad array of issues, and he is feeling better than ever.

A cancer diagnosis and standard treatment create predictable physical and emotional disturbances that can affect long- and short-term quality of life, behavior/coping choices, and immune function, which can subsequently affect outcomes and remission.

Men diagnosed with prostate cancer face a unique set of emotional issues. The diagnosis of cancer itself can be overwhelming enough, but the stigma associated with prostate cancer often prevents them from seeking emotional help. At the time of diagnosis, men can experience a variety of emotions, from fear to anxiety. Studies show that patients mostly fear progression of the disease and the impact it might have on their relationships. Effects of prostate cancer and its treatment on sexual health is the number one concern. Men treated for prostate cancer have described a negative impact of erectile dysfunction on their sense of masculinity and self-esteem. There is often a sense of emasculation and guilt for not being able to have intimate relationships due to anxiety and fear. Patients with loss of libido and erectile dysfunction are at increased risk of depression, fatigue, anxiety, and irritability. Reduced sexual interest can also result in withdrawal of emotional and physical intimacy and can result in a great deal of stress between the patient and his partner. Changes in arousal and sexual stimuli and reduced sexual satisfaction are the most frequent complaints described by couples.

Physical effects of hormone therapy include loss of muscle and bone mass, redistribution of fat, obesity, and increased risk of developing diabetes. These can lead to high-risk health effects such as metabolic syndrome, cardiovascular disease, depression, and anxiety, all of which can affect remission rates and quality of life. In addition, resulting pain from treatment, in and of itself, can cause depressive symptoms and changes in emotional states. Weakness and fatigue caused by the illness, hormones, steroids, and other cancer-related medications can be frustrating and upsetting to independent men who are now dependent on doctors, family, or caretakers.

Men can respond in many ways to being diagnosed, being treated, and living with prostate cancer. They can feel a wide range of emotions. All of these are normal responses. Here are some of the most frequently reported psychological responses:

- *Shock, fear, or anger.* You can feel one or all of these. You might ask yourself: Why me? How did this happen? What did I do, or not do, to cause this to have happened? Other questions might be: What will happen to me, and/or my family and relationship?

- *Denial.* You might feel, initially, like the results are mistaken, or that the technology is not good enough to have definitively diagnosed you. You also might be apt to seek out unconventional information on the Internet. Many men diagnosed with prostate cancer do not have symptoms. It is easier to be in denial when you are asymptomatic.

- *Frustration and disappointment.* A diagnosis and the loss of self-control can lead to a lot of frustration and disappointment with one's self. Many men tend to blame themselves and reflect on their lives and their previous choices.

- *Stress.* Fear of the unknown, the side effects and outcome of treatment can lead to stress and anxiety.

- *Sense of loss.* As men are treated, and/or as the cancer progresses, side effects can create changes in weight, muscle mass, and sexual function and can cause bone loss. These sudden changes can be perceived as loss by many men.

- *Changing identity.* Men's identities incorporate their appearance, activity, sexual drive, and relationships to a great extent. Sudden changes in these can lead to a redefinition of individuals. This can lead to a great deal of anxiety, depression, and confusion.

- *Mood swings.* Different therapies, especially hormone therapy, can cause irritability, hot flashes, and other emotional changes. This can be a rather troublesome symptom for men.

- *Anxiety.* This perhaps is the most common psychological disturbance. Anxiety results from diagnosis through to treatment and to recovery. From diagnosis to recovery, patients worry about side effects from treatment. At recovery, patients worry about the cancer coming back.

- *Feeling alone.* Men often feel isolated after a cancer diagnosis. Often not sharing the diagnosis openly or seeking counseling leads to greater feelings of being alone.

With professional help or direction, these feelings improve or go away. Though it might feel uncomfortable, it is of vital importance that these stressors be recognized and addressed. Stress of this sort has been shown to lead to later presentations of cancer, decreased medical compliance, and increased development of additional illnesses. Increase in psychological stress may increase blood levels of epinephrine and norepinephrine, resulting in increased heart rate, increased blood pressure, and blood sugar levels, which can predispose you to developing diabetes, metabolic syndrome, and put you at a higher risk of developing cancer or recurrence.

EFFECTS ON YOUR IMMUNE SYSTEM

I prioritize optimizing immune function as my number one focus for all patients that visit me, and therefore stress, external or internal, is quite often the culprit that I seek to tame.

During every first office call I ask each patient what they would like to get out of the appointment with me, and then I verbally compare and complement what my objectives are: to decrease side effects, increase quality of life, and ultimately help the immune system to rebound and optimally function. I cannot stress how important robust immune cells are in fighting cancer.

All immune cells play a role in the fight against cancer, but four in particular must be working well. These cells are natural killer (NK) cells, macrophages, CD8 cells, and T helper 1 cells. Normally, these circulate in every person, and remove precancerous and cancer cells. They can be overwhelmed or suppressed by various factors, including external and internal stressors, and even cancer treatment. My plans are always geared to support the immune system during and after cancer treatment to increase quality of life and promote remission.

So, let us take a general look at what happens to the immune system when we are stressed. When we are stressed, one of the main and more significant things that happens is that there is an elevation of the stress hormone cortisol. This is one of the hormones secreted by the adrenal gland involved in the "fight-or-flight" mechanism. Other hormones include adrenaline and epinephrine. In the presence of these hormones, especially when these are secreted chronically, the immune system's ability to fight off antigens and cancer is suppressed. Chronic suppression leaves the body vulnerable to cancer, but also to infection and to other disease processes.

Stress can also have an indirect effect on the immune system as a person may use unhealthy behavioral coping strategies to reduce their stress, such as drinking and smoking. This is extremely common. Alcohol and smoking are known to increase inflammatory processes and deplete vital nutrients needed by the immune system to function.

Inflammation is necessary for short-term responses to illnesses and injuries for eliminating viruses and initiating healing, but chronic inflammation causes less than optimal functioning of the immune system and increases risk for chronic diseases.

Chronic stress can also activate latent viruses such as those associated with cold sores and shingles. When the immune system is depressed, we see an increase in these chronic viral infections surfacing.

High and chronic stress levels also can cause depression and anxiety, again leading to higher levels of inflammation. Sustained high levels of inflammation lead to an overworked, over-tired immune system that cannot properly protect you.

The creation or exacerbation of additional illnesses when you are dealing with cancer also puts a burden on your immune system. Psychological stress is involved in altered immune functioning in many diseases. Altered immune function can cause symptoms of both physical and psychological illnesses. For example, in irritable bowel syndrome, high levels of cortisol can create an increase or exacerbation of gastrointestinal symptoms.

Chronic stress has been shown to increase the risk of developing autoimmune disease, like rheumatoid arthritis, lupus, and Sjogren's. People with autoimmune disease also appear to have difficulty balancing immune responses after exposure to stressors.

Overall, the immune system must be tended to so that the best outcome and remission are achieved. Using a variety of therapies to decrease stress works well for most patients.

I was angry. I am an athlete, I eat right and this shouldn't have happened to me. I was most angry at all the information that told me that I was doing the right thing to be healthy and I still developed prostate cancer. All this made me take a closer look at my life though. While I ate great and exercised, I had a lot of stress, and I did not give sleep the priority. I ended up adding some mind body therapies that are in the same camp as biofeedback to help me understand when I am stressing out.

—*S. S.*

CHAPTER 3

Nurturing Through Nutrients: Easy, Flavorful Recipes

Only I can change my life. No one can do it for me.

—*Carol Burnett*

Now we get to my favorite part of any resource: the solutions!

The goal of the recipes in this book are to aid in:

- Preventing metabolic syndrome
- Balancing blood sugar levels
- Reducing inflammation

What we know from studies is that patients receiving nutritional counseling before, during, and after cancer treatment have better outcomes, quality of life, and experience significantly fewer side effects.

This chapter is essentially a mini cookbook with recipes helpful during cancer treatment and beyond.

Many of the side effects caused by conventional cancer treatment are rooted in preexisting nutritional deficits and increased nutritional needs caused by these therapies. Common nutritional deficiencies include magnesium, calcium, potassium, and sodium. A deficiency in magnesium, for example, can create or exacerbate elevated or depressed blood pressure, muscle cramps, sleep disorders or problems with metabolism. Another common side effect of all therapies is fatigue. Fatigue in patients results from an increased turnover of protein, increased nutrient demand for repair, and disturbances associated with fatty acid metabolism. Proper protein supplementation can substantially decrease treatment-related fatigue and tissue recovery.

Recent research studies have determined that nutrition matters during and after treatment. Therapeutic foods can decrease the side effects of conventional cancer treatment, increase quality of life, and increase remission chances. Knowledge of those foods having negative interactions is also vital.

A LITTLE HOUSEKEEPING

The recipes in this book are made with ingredients that are anti-inflammatory, have a low glycemic index, and are nutrient/mineral dense. And they are delicious! When applying my culinary nutrition expertise during cancer treatment, my goal is to help patients achieve an 80% compliance rate with their diet choices. Some things that I have learned:

1. People are tied closely to their tastes and habits with food

2. Small reasonable changes to diet work better than grand sweeping changes

3. Taste and texture matter, and they especially matter during cancer treatment

In other words, do not "mess" with food unless recipes are going to be flavorful, something recognizable, and easy to make. The good news is that cooking with anti-inflammatory ingredients can encompass all these goals easily. For the most part, and this is thanks to the abundance of different types of food on the planet, many of us already have incorporated eating in a healthy and helpful fashion during cancer care.

Understanding why it is important to eat an anti-inflammatory diet is helpful to compliance. The National Cancer Institute continuously updates its database on several aspects affecting cancer remission and prevention. Many of these recommendations are specific, like reducing intake of red meat to three servings per week. These findings and others are based on nutritional contents of foods that we consume and their inflammatory affects. For example, both cow dairy and red meat contain a higher amount of something called omega-9 fatty acids. These are not "bad" fats per say, but if we consume too many of them, we can tip the balance toward inflammation in our bodies. Inflammation can create damage and reactions that beget more inflammation, causing the cycle to continue. When the damage caused by inflammation exceeds the body's ability to "clean" it up, we begin to get damage at a cellular level. Damaged cells can turn into cancer.

Another example of the importance of eating an anti-inflammatory, whole foods diet has to do with insulin sensitivity. Many people mistakenly attribute sugar as being the culprit in feeding cancer cells. This is not entirely correct. It is the insulin surges that are related to some solid tumors' aggressive growth. Insulin is a hormone that is secreted in response to glucose (aka sugar) levels in the blood stream. Insulin presence signals to the cells to grow and divide. Normal cells consume the glucose at a normal rate, divide, and then have a mechanism to turn themselves off. Some solid tumor cells, research shows, more aggressively take up glucose, given the signal by insulin, and they do not contain the mechanism to turn off growth or slow down growth. Eating a diet containing complex carbohydrates and whole foods causes the blood sugar and insulin levels to maintain a steady state; that is, no big ups or downs in insulin. Eating this way with whole foods is the foundation of an anti-inflammatory diet.

The easiest way to adhere to an anti-inflammatory diet is first to be conscious of what you are eating. Take a week or two to just assess what you are eating:

- How many boxed and processed foods am I eating?
- How many times a week am I eating out and what kinds of foods am I eating?
- How much processed sugar and simple carbohydrates am I eating per day?
- How many whole foods do I have in my diet?

Once you have assessed this, make steps to trade out one thing at a time. For example, maybe you eat lunch out at a fast food restaurant five times a week. The first step could be that you eat out four times a week and bring a healthy meal from home once per week. Or you could choose to eat at a healthier venue that offers lean meats, salads, and healthy soup options. Small changes, for many, add up to long-term compliance.

Of course, some people are very successful in making a 180-degree change in their diet once diagnosed with cancer. That is okay as well.

SUGGESTIONS FOR YOUR PANTRY

I would suggest decreasing or eliminating the following foods from your pantry and refrigerator:

Wheat flour	Corn
Corn meal	Soy oil
White sugar	Canola oil
Brown sugar	Cow's milk and cheeses
Agave syrup	Soda
Margarine	Fruit juice
White potatoes	Alcohol

Think about replacing these with:

Barley flour	Vinegar
Almond flour	Herbs and spices (e.g., rosemary,
Oat flour	cumin, ginger)
Ground flaxseeds	Extra virgin olive oil
Goat cheese	Coconut oil
Sheep cheese	Walnuts
Butter or ghee	

These foods are readily available at most grocery stores. In addition, you can find them online.

Wherever you are in the process of dietary changes, know that diet and nutrition do make a difference in treatment side effects and outcome. An anti-inflammatory diet can make a difference, and you can still enjoy your meals with the side benefit of having increased amount of energy and protection.

Use these recipes as starting points. Add a side dish or two to one of your favorite meals. Try to integrate these recipes slowly so it is not quite a jolt to your regular patterns. For more recipes ideas, check out my blog at www.drlisapricend.com.

Let us dive into the nitty gritty and start making meal plans, shall we?

MORNING DISHES

SWEET POTATO AND VEGGIE PANCAKES

Who does not love the comfort of a potato pancake? Slightly different from the usual, this recipe uses sweet potatoes and a variety of scrumptious fresh herbs to create a delightful and filling meal.

Ingredients:

1 cup chickpea flour

1 teaspoon turmeric powder

1 cup water

⅓ cup cooked mashed sweet potato

1 cup cilantro, finely chopped

1 cup parsnips, grated

1 cup cooked beet greens, chopped (slightly wilted, from 4 cups fresh)

Salt to taste

Oil for cooking

You may want to adjust the water to alter the consistency.

Directions:

In a large bowl, mix together flour, spices, sweet potato; beat in greens and parsnips and water. Turn oven to low, about 200°F (95°C). You will place the cooked pancakes in the oven until you are ready to serve. Heat oil in the bottom of a heavy skillet over medium high heat.

Press a heaping tablespoon of the mixture flat, then place it into the skillet. Cook until browned on both sides which should take about 8 to 10 minutes. Transfer to oven-proof dish and into the oven as you cook the rest of the pancakes.

Makes 4 servings.

NUTRITIONAL ANALYSIS PER SERVING:

Calories—162	Protein—6.61 g	Magnesium—70 mg	Omega-6—0.682 g
Total Fat—1.81 g	Iron—2.02 mg	Potassium—599 mg	Folate—151 mcg
Carbohydrates—30.61 g	Sodium—52 mg	Vitamin C—18.7 mg	
Dietary Fiber—6.9 g	Calcium—55 mg	Omega-3—0.026 g	

This recipe contains a good amount of vitamins A and K and manganese. These vitamins are important for tissue repair and healthy blood cells.

QUINOA MORNING CEREAL

This is one of my favorite meals as an alternative to cold cereal or oatmeal in the morning. The flavor of quinoa is nutty, and the texture is mildly chewy. Quinoa is a versatile grain and can be prepared several ways.

Ingredients:

1 cup quinoa, cooked

1 tbs cinnamon

1 tbs honey

¼ cup walnuts

½ pear, fresh, ripe, diced

Directions:

Rinse the quinoa with cold water. Add two cups of water to a pot and add quinoa.

Place over a medium heat and bring to a boil. Reduce to a simmer for 10 to 15 minutes, or until the quinoa is tender and the liquid is absorbed. Turn the heat off, and add cinnamon, honey, walnuts, and pear. Enjoy.

Makes 4 servings.

NUTRITIONAL ANALYSIS PER SERVING:

Calories—231	Protein—15 g	Magnesium—145 mg	Omega-6—8.1g
Total Fat—15 g	Iron—4.5 mg	Potassium—602 mg	Folate—170 mcg
Carbohydrates—71 g	Sodium—5.5 mg	Vitamin C—1.5 mg	
Dietary Fiber—10.2 g	Calcium—80 mg	Omega-3—1.5 g	

This recipe contains good levels of a number of branched chained amino acids preferred by the immune system and gut cells as energy sources. It also is an excellent source of protein and omega-3 fatty acids.

OATMEAL PANCAKES

Simple and easy, this pancake is quick to make in the morning. These healthy pancakes are satisfying and flavorful. You will love the comforting blend of vanilla, cinnamon, and honey in the morning.

Ingredients:

1 cup oatmeal, cooked

½ cup coconut milk

1 banana, mashed

2 tbs flaxseeds, soaked (¼ cup of water)

1 to 2 tbs vanilla extract

1 tsp cinnamon

1 tbs honey

Pinch of salt

Oil for cooking

Directions:

In a bowl, mix all the ingredients. Heat a griddle or pan and add a heaping tablespoon of the mixture and flattened it. Let the pancake brown. Gently flip and let thoroughly cook through, about 1 to 2 minutes.

Makes 4 servings.

NUTRITIONAL ANALYSIS PER SERVING:

Calories—371	Protein—5.1 g	Magnesium—86 mg	Omega-6—0.6 g
Total Fat—18.7 g	Iron—1.5 mg	Potassium—415 mg	Folate—24 mcg
Carbohydrates—44 g	Sodium—71 mg	Vitamin C—5.3 mg	
Dietary Fiber—7.25 g	Calcium—55 mg	Omega-3—2.35 g	

This recipe is particularly a good source of vitamin B1 and manganese.

BUFFALO HASH

This dish has everything. It provides an assortment of textures and flavors. Buffalo meat is rich in flavor, and slightly sweet. It combines well with curry spice, and the earthy tones of the cruciferous vegetables in this recipe.

Ingredients:

3 ounces of buffalo meat

½ cup cauliflower, chopped

½ cup broccoli, chopped

4 cloves of garlic, minced

½ red pepper, sliced, seeds removed

1 tsp curry powder

1 tsp cumin

4 eggs

1 tbs olive oil

Directions:

In a skillet over medium heat, brown the buffalo meat. In the same skillet, add oil, vegetables, garlic, cumin, and curry powder. Mix. Turn the heat to high and quickly sauté the mixture until the vegetables are soft and slightly browned, about 4 to 5 minutes. Turn heat off and cover to retain heat.

In another pan, add oil and cook eggs sunny side up to preferred consistency.

Place meat and vegetables on a plate and place the egg on top of the mixture. Salt to taste.

Makes 4 servings.

NUTRITIONAL ANALYSIS PER SERVING:

Calories—285	Protein—23.49 g	Magnesium—114 mg	Omega-6—1.4 g
Total Fat—12.78 g	Iron—7.34 mg	Potassium—1,060 mg	Folate—132 mcg
Carbohydrates—22.23 g	Sodium—83 mg	Vitamin C—3 mg	
Dietary Fiber—9.2 g	Calcium—156 mg	Omega-3—0.117 g	

This recipe contains a good source of tryptophan and several other branched chain amino acids, and vitamins B_2, B_3, B_{12}, and B_6. Tryptophan is an amino acid that is needed to make the "feel good" neurotransmitter serotonin.

MORNING BURRITOS

This is a fantastic flavorful recipe that provides a great amount of protein to start the day. There are a variety of herbs and textures blended to create an easily assembled morning meal.

Ingredients:

4 spelt tortillas

1 tbs extra virgin olive oil

¼ cup chopped green onions

1 ripe tomato, chopped

2 cups cilantro, chopped

1 lime (juice from)

½ tsp chili powder

1 cup black beans, cooked (or from a can)

4 eggs

½ cup vegan sour cream

1 ½ cups chopped fresh spinach

½ tsp salt

¼ tsp black pepper

Directions:

In a large skillet, heat oil over medium heat. Add green onions and spinach and cook for about 1 minute. Add black beans, chili powder, salt and pepper and cook for an additional 5 minutes.

Mix tomato, cilantro, and juice from one lime and a pinch of salt. Toss gently.

Scramble eggs and add salt and pepper to taste.

Per tortilla, layer ¼ of the black bean mixture, ¼ of the tomato and ¼ of the scrambled eggs. Top with two tbs of sour cream.

Makes 4 servings.

NUTRITIONAL ANALYSIS PER SERVING:

Calories—514	Protein—26.11 g	Magnesium—124 mg	Omega-6—1.1g
Total Fat—18.87 g	Iron—7.33 mg	Potassium—1,212 mg	Folate—403 mcg
Carbohydrates—60.69 g	Sodium—545 mg	Vitamin C—137 mg	
Dietary Fiber—9.8 g	Calcium—230 mg	Omega-3—0.3 g	

This recipe is a good source of protein and vitamins B_{12}, B_1, A, and K.

SAVORY OATMEAL WITH EGG

Yes, it is true, oatmeal can be savory and delicious. This recipe combines a variety of fragrant herbs and vegetables plus a favorite comfort food, a fried egg. It is a pleasant departure from your regular sweet oatmeal.

Ingredients:

¼ cup steel cut oats (quick cooking)

¾ cup of water

1 tbs flaxseeds, ground

1 tsp turmeric, grated

¼ cup green onions, chopped

1 tbs onion, chopped

¼ cup red bell pepper

2 tbs extra virgin olive oil

1 large egg

Salt and pepper to taste

Directions:

In a pot, add water and bring to a boil. Add oatmeal and cook for about 5 minutes. You will know it is done when the oatmeal is thickened and very little water is left. Turn off heat and stir in the flaxseeds. Add oatmeal to a bowl.

In a skillet, add one tbs of the olive oil over medium heat. Add onions, bell peppers, and turmeric, and salt and pepper to taste. Place veggies over oatmeal in the bowl.

In a skillet, add the remaining one tbs of olive oil and heat over a medium to high flame. Fry the egg to preferred consistency and add to the top of the oatmeal and vegetable mixture.

Makes 1 serving.

NUTRITIONAL ANALYSIS PER SERVING:

Calories—276	Protein—7.14 g	Magnesium—80 mg	Omega-6—2.0 g
Total Fat—23.1 g	Iron—3.5 mg	Potassium—307 mg	Folate—55 mcg
Carbohydrates—15.2 g	Sodium—20 mg	Vitamin C—32.6 mg	
Dietary Fiber—5.9 g	Calcium—90 mg	Omega-3—2.5 g	

This recipe contains a good source of omega-3 fatty acid and vitamin A. These two nutrients are important in anti-inflammatory processes, and in tissue healing.

MAIN DISHES

TURKEY ROLL UP

No, it is not Thanksgiving, but you will think it is when eating this festive roll up. With cranberries and all, this zesty dish has notes of sweet and warm flavors. This roll up provides a good amount of zinc and magnesium.

Ingredients:

1 cup of turkey, dark meat, roasted and shredded

¼ cup of dried cranberries

1 to 2 tbs of aioli

1 tbs parsley, minced

2 tbs extra virgin olive oil

¼ cup of Brussels sprouts, thinly cut and sautéed

1 to 2 pinches of salt

1 spelt or rice tortilla

Directions:

Add extra virgin olive oil to a skillet and sauté Brussels sprouts until slightly browned and crispy. Add salt to taste.

To a bowl, add turkey meat, cranberries, aioli, and parsley. Mix and toss. Place cooked Brussels sprouts on tortilla, and turkey mixture on top. Fold or roll up the tortilla. Enjoy.

Makes 1 serving.

NUTRITIONAL ANALYSIS PER SERVING:

Calories—641	Protein—16 g	Magnesium—36 mg	Omega-6—4.8 g
Total Fat—48.27 g	Iron—3.71 mg	Potassium—342 mg	Folate—84 mcg
Carbohydrates—35.28 g	Sodium—499 mg	Vitamin C—50.5 mg	
Dietary Fiber—2.3 g	Calcium—208 mg	Omega-3—0.5 g	

This recipe contains a good amount of selenium and vitamin K. Selenium is an important anti-oxidant for men's prostate health.

MUSSELS WITH WHITE WINE AND THYME

There is an ease involved in making this dish that does not match its delicious flavor. The meal mixes earthy notes of fresh herbs and wine blended to perfection. The resulting broth, infused with fresh thyme and parsley, is great for dipping a hearty homemade sourdough bread.

Ingredients:

2 pounds of mussels

2 tbs ghee or butter

¼ cup minced scallions

1 tbs fresh thyme

1 tbs minced garlic

¼ cup of parsley

1 cup of white wine

Directions:

Clean mussels by scrubbing with a brush under cool water. Discard any that are opened. Set clean mussels aside.

In a skillet, sauté scallions, garlic, and ghee for 5 minutes or until slightly browned. Add 1 cup of white wine and allow to simmer for 5 to 10 minutes. Add mussels, cover skillet, and cook until mussels open. Stir in fresh thyme and parsley. Enjoy.

Makes 4 servings.

NUTRITIONAL ANALYSIS PER SERVING:

Calories—241	Protein—27.9 g	Magnesium—88 mg	Omega-6—0.2 g
Total Fat—9 g	Iron—9.73 mg	Potassium—832 mg	Folate—106 mcg
Carbohydrates—10.5 g	Sodium—688 mg	Vitamin C—25.9 mg	
Dietary Fiber—1.2 g	Calcium—83 mg	Omega-3—1.1 g	

This recipe contains an excellent amount of omega-3 fatty acids, branched chained amino acids, selenium, manganese, and vitamins K and B[12].

VEGETABLE FRITTERS

These crispy fritters are spicy and pack a healthy punch. They contain a colorful array of vegetables and are sure to be the perfect comfort food. Eat them as a snack or as a side dish with an entrée.

Ingredients:

2 cups raw veggies, grated and blended (broccoli, cauliflower, carrots, asparagus)

¼ cup grated onions

1 cup garbanzo bean or oat flour

1 tsp baking powder

½ tsp salt

¼ tsp turmeric

¼ tsp cayenne

¼ cup tahini

⅛ tsp black pepper

1 cup unsweetened coconut or hemp milk

Extra virgin olive oil (¼ inch in pan or skillet)

Directions:

To a bowl, add milk, tahini, onions, flour, baking powder, salt, turmeric, cayenne, and black pepper. Mix. Add the grated vegetables and fold into the mixture. Heat oil in skillet and drop a tablespoon of mixture into the pan. Brown the fritters and serve immediately.

Makes 4 servings.

NUTRITIONAL ANALYSIS PER SERVING:

Calories—290	Protein—7.5 g	Magnesium—30 mg	Omega-6—4.1 g
Total Fat—16.25 g	Iron—3.41 mg	Potassium—315 mg	Folate—91 mcg
Carbohydrates—30.42 g	Sodium—330 mg	Vitamin C—4.6 mg	
Dietary Fiber—3 g	Calcium—181 mg	Omega-3—0.1 g	

This recipe contains a good amount of vitamin K.

BROCCOLI, BLACK BEANS, AND WALNUTS OVER ROASTED SWEET POTATOES

This is a convenient and easy to make all-in-one meal that is packed with protein, fiber, and essential omega-3 fatty acids. A wholesome and filling dish, you might find the flavor combination addicting.

Ingredients:

4 cups broccoli florets, chopped

2 tbs extra virgin olive oil

1 cup canned black beans

2 tbs chopped walnuts

2 tbs chopped parsley

2 sweet potatoes, uncooked, ¼ to ½ inch slices

Salt and pepper to taste

2 garlic cloves

2 green onions

Directions:

Heat oven to 450 degrees and place sliced sweet potatoes in baking dish. Brush withoil and add salt and pepper. Cook for 18 to 22 minutes. While they are cooking, prepare your bean mixture.

To a pot, add black beans with juice from the can, broccoli, garlic, green onions, walnuts, and parsley. Heat mixture over medium heat until broccoli florets are soft, about 8 to 10 minutes.

Remove sweet potatoes from the oven. They should be soft. Place slices on plates and spoon black bean mixture over the sliced sweet potato. Enjoy.

Makes 4 servings.

NUTRITIONAL ANALYSIS PER SERVING:

Calories—208	Protein—7.0 g	Magnesium—56 mg	Omega-6—2.0 g
Total Fat—9.52 g	Iron—2.7 mg	Potassium—529 mg	Folate—83 mcg
Carbohydrates—25.48 g	Sodium—529 mg	Vitamin C—15.1 mg	
Dietary Fiber—7.6 g	Calcium—95 mg	Omega-3—0.2 g	

This recipe supplies an excellent amount of vitamins A and K.

WHITE BEAN SOUP

I love how easy this lunch or dinner recipe is. A bowlful is filling and satisfying. Cooked to perfection, this soup is creamy and savory with flavor notes from the Southwest.

Ingredients:

3 cups of cooked white beans

3 cups of vegetable broth

2 tbs lime juice

2 tbs minced fresh basil

2 tbs minced fresh cilantro

2 tbs olive oil

1 medium onion sliced

3 cloves minced garlic

Salt to taste

Directions:

In a skillet, heat the olive oil and sauté the onions for about 10 to 15 minutes. Add beans and minced garlic. Simmer for 15 minutes. Stir in broth and salt to taste and simmer for 15 more minutes.

Pour the mixture into a blender and puree it. Pour the mixture into a pot and simmer over medium heat until hot. Add lime juice, basil, and cilantro. Stir. Serve and enjoy.

Makes 4 servings.

NUTRITIONAL ANALYSIS PER SERVING:

Calories—271	Protein—13.6 g	Magnesium—89 mg	Omega-6—0.8 g
Total Fat—7.27 g	Iron—5.16 mg	Potassium—813 mg	Folate—116 mcg
Carbohydrates—39.6 g	Sodium—422 mg	Vitamin C—4.2 mg	
Dietary Fiber—9 g	Calcium—134 mg	Omega-3—0.15 g	

This recip contains a good source of tryptophan, phenylalanine, and tyrosine, all amino acids involved in sleep and mental wellness. It also contains a good source of manganese.

LENTILS WITH LEEKS AND WILD MUSHROOMS

I love lentils. They are easy and fast to make and can be seasoned many different ways. Lentils are also more easily digested than beans, while still providing a good amount of protein. This recipe is an homage to the Pacific Northwest in the fall with its Chanterelles and other spices.

Ingredients:

2 cups lentils

4 cups of water

4 carrots, sliced

1 bulb of garlic, minced

1 leek, sliced

1 sweet potato, diced

4 medium-sized Chanterelles (or 2 cups of shiitake mushrooms)

¼ cup tamari

1 tsp cumin

Directions:

Place 4 cups of water into a pot and add the lentils and the diced sweet potatoes. Heat over medium heat for 15 to 20 minutes. Turn the heat down to simmer and add the carrots, garlic, leek, mushrooms, cumin, and tamari. Cook for an additional 30 to 40 minutes. Add salt to taste.

Makes 4 servings.

NUTRITIONAL ANALYSIS PER SERVING:

Calories—147	Protein—8 g	Magnesium—53 mg	Omega-6—0.4 g
Total Fat—1.0 g	Iron—4.6 mg	Potassium—682 mg	Folate—71 mcg
Carbohydrates—30.5 g	Sodium—1,073 mg	Vitamin C—20.2 mg	
Dietary Fiber—5.1 g	Calcium—90 mg	Omega-3—0.03 g	

This recipe contains a good source of vitamins A and K, copper, and manganese.

ZUCCHINI PASTA WITH CASHEWS AND GROUND FLAXSEEDS

This dish is light with a rich taste. It is the perfect alternative to pasta. The zucchini absorbs the flavors of garlic and basil while keeping its crisp texture.

Ingredients:

2 large zucchinis sliced into spaghetti-like strands

1 cup of fresh basil, chopped

½ cup of extra virgin olive oil

2 to 3 tbs minced garlic

½ cup of cashews

½ tbs of ground flaxseeds

Directions:

Slice the zucchinis into long strips. Add two tbs of the olive oil and minced garlic to a pan and heat. Add zucchini strips and cook for 5 to 7 minutes on medium. Turn the heat off. To a blender, add chopped basil, cashews, flaxseeds, and olive oil. Mix and immediately add to pan with zucchini strips. Serve and enjoy.

Makes 4 servings.

NUTRITIONAL ANALYSIS PER SERVING:

Calories—526	Protein—10.2 g	Magnesium—159 mg	Omega-6—6.3 g
Total Fat—48 g	Iron—4 mg	Potassium—460 mg	Folate—26 mcg
Carbohydrates—19.2 g	Sodium—6 mg	Vitamin C—10.1 mg	
Dietary Fiber—3.4 g	Calcium—76 mg	Omega-3—1.5 g	

Flaxseeds contain a good amount of omega-3 fatty acid, which are anti-inflammatory and also aid in tissue regeneration. In addition, they contain soluble fiber which adds bulking and aids in proper bowel function. Flaxseeds contain a component called lignan that has been shown to have helpful effects for gut flora and gut cells. This recipe contains a good source of the amino acid tryptophan, copper, manganese, and vitamin K.

STUFFED AVOCADOS

How great are avocados, you might ask? They are almost perfect. In this recipe, they live up to the rating. This meal is actually in the avocado. It is easy to make, buttery, and satisfyingly good.

Ingredients:

1 avocado

1 can cooked salmon

½ cup cilantro, chopped

2 cloves garlic, minced

¼ onion, finely chopped

½ lemon, juice from

1 tsp aioli

1 celery stalk, chopped

Directions:

Empty the can of salmon into a bowl. Add garlic, onion, aioli, celery, cilantro, and lemon juice. Mix. Slice an avocado in half. Remove the seed. Divide and add mixture where the seed had been. Enjoy.

Makes 4 servings.

NUTRITIONAL ANALYSIS PER SERVING:

Calories—501	Protein—45.72 g	Magnesium—99 mg	Omega-6—2.4 g
Total Fat—25.7 g	Iron—1.95 mg	Potassium—1,259 mg	Folate—92 mcg
Carbohydrates—11.5 g	Sodium—944 mg	Vitamin C—13 mg	
Dietary Fiber—7.4 g	Calcium—446 mg	Omega-3—3.1 g	

This recipe contains a good amount of tryptophan and other branched chain amino acids, as well as vitamins B_3, B_6, B_{12}, and D, and selenium.

ELK QUESADILLA

Game meats are excellent sources of lean protein. Elk can be a wonderful alternative in quesadilla, and it is flavorful and has a very clean taste. It is very tender and does not need marinating.

Ingredients:

1 tbs olive oil

¼ onion, chopped

½ red bell pepper, sliced

2 tbs fresh basil, chopped

3 ounces elk, cut into bite-sized pieces

1 tsp cumin

Salt and pepper to taste

1 spelt tortilla

Option: If you cannot find elk, you can substitute beef or bison meat.

Directions:

In a skillet over medium heat, olive oil and sauté onions and peppers until slightly soft. Raise heat to medium high, add the elk. Sauté elk and vegetables, basil, and cumin for about 5 to 8 minutes in a covered pan or until browned. Watch that the elk does not dry out.

Warm a tortilla in the oven or use at room temperature. Place vegetable and elk mixture on the tortilla and fold over. Enjoy.

Makes 1 serving.

NUTRITIONAL ANALYSIS PER SERVING:

Calories—465	Protein—24.67 g	Magnesium—56 mg	Omega-6—2.12 g
Total Fat—20.8 g	Iron—10.4 mg	Potassium—539 mg	Folate—103 mcg
Carbohydrates—45.7 g	Sodium—393 mg	Vitamin C—35.5 mg	
Dietary Fiber—3.5 g	Calcium—70 mg	Omega-3—0.1 g	

This recipe is a great source of protein and especially branched chain amino acid, as well as vitamins B_{12}, B_1, B_3, and B_6.

SALMON WITH BASIL AND APRICOTS

If you like fish dishes, you will love this one. A medley of ingredients creates a delightful and interesting flavor sensations. The essential oils from basil and fennel create a lingering yet subtle taste experience.

Ingredients:

8 ounces of salmon, fillet

1 can of coconut milk

1 cup fresh basil, chopped

2 fennel bulbs, fresh, sliced

¼ cup chopped, dried apricots

2 lemons, juiced

1 tsp salt

Pepper to taste

Directions:

Heat the oven to a temperature of 425 degrees. Line the bottom of an iron skillet or casserole dish with the sliced fennel. Place the salmon on top of the fennel. Poke fork holes along the salmon fillet. Add the lemon juice to the fish and also the salt and pepper. Pour the can of coconut milk into a bowl. Add apricots and basil to the coconut milk and mix. Pour coconut milk mixture over fish. Cook for 20 to 30 minutes or until fish flakes.

Makes 4 servings.

NUTRITIONAL ANALYSIS PER SERVING:

Calories—267	Protein—14.3 g	Magnesium—57 mg	Omega-6—0.2 g
Total Fat—18.6 g	Iron—2.2 mg	Potassium—714 mg	Folate—33 mcg
Carbohydrates—13.9 g	Sodium—868 mg	Vitamin C—15.8 mg	
Dietary Fiber—3.9 g	Calcium—167 mg	Omega-3—0.8 g	

This recipe contains a good source of branched chained amino acids and vitamins A, D, and K.

QUINOA, STEAK, AND MIXED VEGETABLE SAUTÉ

According to studies, plant-based diets are best for cancer patients with the use of small amounts of meat primarily used as a condiment to flavor food rather than the main event. This satisfying recipe keeps to that order. The flavor can be described as down home and earthy.

Ingredients:

6 ounces of steak, free range, hormone-free

1 cup quinoa

2 cups water

1 tbs extra virgin olive oil

½ small red onion

½ medium red bell pepper, chopped

½ medium zucchini, chopped

½ cup shiitake mushrooms, chopped

1 tomato, chopped

3 tbs parsley, chopped

Salt and pepper to taste

Directions:

Put water in a pot and bring to a boil. Add the quinoa and reduce the heat to medium. Cook for 20 to 30 minutes until water is mostly gone. Remove from heat.

In a skillet, add oil and onion, pepper, zucchini, mushrooms, and tomato. Cook over medium heat until vegetables are soft, which will take about 10 minutes. Mix well with quinoa.

Heat a skillet over a high flame. If you have a lean piece of meat you may need a small amount of olive oil to cook the beef. Add the steak to the skillet and cover. Cook over high flame for 3 to 4 minutes. Flip the steak and cook for another 3 to 4 minutes. The steak should be slightly pink inside. Salt and pepper to taste. Remove from skillet and cut into thin slices and add to the quinoa mixture or eat separately.

Makes 4 servings.

NUTRITIONAL ANALYSIS PER SERVING:

Calories—572	Protein—36.9 g	Magnesium—198 mg	Omega-6—3.3 g
Total Fat—20.8 g	Iron—6.6 mg	Potassium—968 mg	Folate—186 mcg
Carbohydrates—60.7 g	Sodium—364 mg	Vitamin C—45.5 mg	
Dietary Fiber—7.5 g	Calcium—99 mg	Omega-3—0.3 g	

This recipe contains a great amount of protein and vitamins B_6, K, A, and B_{12}. It also contains a good amount of minerals.

PAN-SEARED BEEF WITH ARTICHOKES AND OLIVES

This recipe is an excellent source of protein. It has a slightly salty taste without having a high sodium content and is very fragrant.

Ingredients:

6 ounces of steak, free-range, hormone-free

2 tbs olive oil

2 cloves garlic, minced

1 can tomatoes, diced, drained

1 cup artichoke hearts, cut into slices

¼ cup black olives

1 tsp capers

2 tbs parsley, chopped

Salt and pepper to taste

Optional: If you can find bison steaks, you may substitute for beef.

Directions:

In a skillet, heat 1 tablespoon of the oil over medium heat. Add the garlic and cook for about 30 seconds to 1 minute. Add the tomatoes, artichokes, olives, capers, and parsley. Salt and pepper to taste. Cook for about 5 to 6 minutes.

In another skillet, add 1 tablespoon of olive oil over high heat. Place steak in skillet and cover. Cook for 3 to 4 minutes. Flip the steak and cook for another 3 to 4 minutes. The inside of the meat should have only a slight pink color. If red, cook for a little while longer. Salt and pepper to taste.

Remove meat and place it on a plate. Spoon vegetable mixture over meat. Enjoy.

Can serve over brown rice or quinoa.

Makes 4 servings.

NUTRITIONAL ANALYSIS PER SERVING:

Calories—305	Protein—27.4 g	Magnesium—70 mg	Omega-6—0.9 g
Total Fat—17.3 g	Iron—4.0 mg	Potassium—712 mg	Folate—75 mcg
Carbohydrates—13.4 g	Sodium—654 mg	Vitamin C—24.3 mg	
Dietary Fiber—5.9 g	Calcium—84 mg	Omega-3—0.1 g	

This recipe is high in protein and vitamins B_1, K, and A. It is also a good source of zinc.

SIDE DISHES

COLLARD SLAW

Not your average coleslaw! With a couple of additions, this recipe converts coleslaw to a zippy and healthy recipe that still retains flavor. The addition of cayenne makes this recipe a little spicier than standard. Super easy to make and you will love it.

Ingredients:

2 cups fresh collard greens, sliced finely

2 cups cabbage, sliced finely

1 tsp cayenne

¼ cup sunflower seeds

¼ cup sesame seeds

2 tbs apple cider vinegar

1 tsp honey

1 tbs aioli

Pinch of salt

Directions:

Combine all ingredients in a bowl and let stand for at least 30 minutes to 1 hour before serving. Enjoy.

Makes 4 servings.

NUTRITIONAL ANALYSIS PER SERVING:

Calories—147	Protein—5 g	Magnesium—74 mg	Omega-6—4.8 g
Total Fat—11.2 g	Iron—1.55 mg	Potassium—253 mg	Folate—62 mcg
Carbohydrates—9.5 g	Sodium—39 mg	Vitamin C—32 mg	
Dietary Fiber—3.6 g	Calcium—76 mg	Omega-3—0.1 g	

This recipe contains a good amount of vitamins A and K.

CITRUS-ROASTED ASPARAGUS

Seasoned to perfection, the blended flavors of citrus and nutty are sure to melt in your mouth. Roasting asparagus caramelizes natural sugars, bringing out a slight sweetness and resulting in a tender consistency. You will love this savory side dish.

Ingredients:

1 medium shallot, minced
⅓ cup of fresh lemon juice
¼ cup of orange juice
¼ cup pine nuts
1 tsp of honey
2 tbs of extra virgin olive oil
Salt and pepper to taste
1 lb fresh asparagus, trimmed

Directions:

Preheat oven to 425 degrees. Roast asparagus for about 10 minutes.

In a bowl, mix lemon juice, orange juice, honey, olive oil, and salt and pepper. Mix well. Add to the asparagus along with nuts and minced shallot. Roast for 10 more minutes. Serve. Enjoy.

Makes 4 servings.

NUTRITIONAL ANALYSIS PER SERVING:

Calories—172	Protein—4.4 g	Magnesium—45 mg	Omega-6—3.5 g
Total Fat—12.7 g	Iron—3.2 mg	Potassium—400 mg	Folate—76 mcg
Carbohydrates—13.7 g	Sodium—6 mg	Vitamin C—21.2 mg	
Dietary Fiber—3.5 g	Calcium—40 mg	Omega-3—0.1 g	

This recipe is a good source of vitamin K.

BEET GREENS

This is not your average vegetable side dish! Beet greens are not often prepared as a regular dish. They are delicious and very nutritious. Unlike mustard and kale greens, beet greens have a sweeter and milder flavor. The spices used give the dish a North African flavor. Great gateway green for those who have shied away from greens.

Ingredients:

Greens from 2 bunches of beets (usually 8 beets), chopped

⅓ cup lemon juice

½ cup dried apricots, chopped

½ tsp turmeric

½ tsp crushed red pepper

1–2 tbs extra virgin olive oil

Salt and pepper to taste

Directions:

Heat a skillet with olive oil on medium heat. Add chopped greens, apricots, and spices. Sauté for 2 to 3 minutes. Add lemon juice right at the end of cooking. Salt and pepper to taste. Serve immediately.

Makes 4 servings.

NUTRITIONAL ANALYSIS PER SERVING:

Calories—164	Protein—2.9 g	Magnesium—66 mg	Omega-6—0.7 g
Total Fat—7.11 g	Iron—2.9 mg	Potassium—998 mg	Folate—23 mcg
Carbohydrates—26.4 g	Sodium—176 mg	Vitamin C—38.7 mg	
Dietary Fiber—5.3 g	Calcium—109 mg	Omega-3—0.1 g	

Beet greens are a good source of calcium and potassium.

BEETS WITH WALNUTS, ONIONS, AND GOAT CHEESE

You will love this colorful root salad. Its wonderful combination of natural flavors provides sweet and sour notes, with a crunchy texture.

Ingredients:

8 beets, cubed

¼ cup balsamic vinegar

4 ounces of goat cheese, soft and crumbly

½ cup walnuts, chopped

1 onion, sliced and halved

Pinch of salt

Directions:

Steam the cubed beets for 20 minutes on medium heat. Drain and rinse with cold water. Place beets into a bowl and add onions, salt, and balsamic vinegar. Mix. Add goat cheese and walnuts to the top of the mixture. Serve.

Makes 4 servings.

NUTRITIONAL ANALYSIS PER SERVING:

Calories—198	Protein—9.3 g	Magnesium—47 mg	Omega-6—2.11 g
Total Fat—11.1 g	Iron—1.5 mg	Potassium—395 mg	Folate—91 mcg
Carbohydrates—16.4 g	Sodium—172 mg	Vitamin C—5.7 mg	
Dietary Fiber—2.8 g	Calcium—222 mg	Omega 3—0.5 g	

This recipe contains a good amount of protein and omega-3 and omega-6 fatty acids.

LEMON GLAZED PARSNIPS WITH APRICOTS

A dish with flare. Parsnips are front and center in this nutty and earthy recipe. You might think apricots are added for their flavor, but it is their iron content we are really after. If you are craving a bright, crispy side dish, look no further.

Ingredients:

1 lb parsnips, cut into strips

1 tsp honey

1 tbs ghee or butter

1 tbs lemon juice

½ cup dried apricots, chopped

Directions:

Heat the oven to 400 degrees. Peel the parsnips and trim off both ends and cut into strips. In a separate small pot, add the ghee, honey, lemon, and apricots. Mix well. Place the prepared parsnips in the pot and coat them with the liquid mixture, then place them into a casserole dish. Pour the remaining mixture, including the apricots, into the casserole dish. Roast in the oven for 35 minutes, turning occasionally until golden and tender.

Makes 4 servings.

NUTRITIONAL ANALYSIS PER SERVING:

Calories—156	Protein—2 g	Magnesium—38 mg	Omega-6—0.1 g
Total Fat—3.3 g	Iron—1.1 mg	Potassium—620 mg	Folate—79 mcg
Carbohydrates—32.3 g	Sodium—36 mg	Vitamin C—21 mg	
Dietary Fiber—6.8 g	Calcium—51 mg	Omega-3—0.01 g	

Apricots contain a surprisingly large amount iron. Iron is an important factor in red blood cell development.

WARM BEET AND PEAR SALAD WITH GOAT CHEESE

This sweet and salty salad is served warm. It is sure to be a hit as a side dish or a light snack.

Ingredients:

4 medium beets, fresh

2 pears

4 tbs of balsamic vinegar

1 tbs of extra virgin olive oil

½ cup of goat cheese

Directions:

Quarter beets and place them on an oven pan. Place in oven and cook for 20 minutes.

Slice pears into eight parts and then half the slices. Place in mixing dish. Once beets are done, add them directly to the pears. To this mixture, add vinegar, and olive oil. Serve onto a plate with crumbled goat cheese on top.

Makes 4 servings.

NUTRITIONAL ANALYSIS PER SERVING:

Calories—201	Protein—8.2 g	Magnesium—37 mg	Omega-6—0.5 g
Total Fat—11.2 g	Iron—1.2 mg	Potassium—368 mg	Folate—95 mcg
Carbohydrates—17.5 g	Sodium—158 mg	Vitamin C—6.3 mg	
Dietary Fiber—4.5 g	Calcium—210 mg	Omega-3—0.03 g	

Beets and pears contain soluble fiber that includes inulin and pectin. These provide the gut cells with healthy nutrition and also cause bulking in the colon, which stimulates bowel emptying.

PLUM CHUTNEY

You may want to include this succulent condiment as a staple with your lunch and dinner meals. It is sweet and tangy and helps to bring out the flavors of your favorite foods. This delightful dish contains good levels of vitamin C, iron, and potassium. It is also a good source of soluble fiber.

Ingredients:

8 plums, sliced and halved, skin on, discard pit

1 medium red onion, coarsely chopped

⅓ cup dried currants

¼ cup apple cider vinegar

2 large garlic cloves, cut paper thin

1 tsp mustard seed

½ tsp salt

½ tsp ground black pepper

½ cup water

⅓ cup honey

Directions:

Bring ½ cup of water to a boil. Place plums into pot with boiling water. When it boils again, add all other ingredients. Cook for 25 to 30 minutes until most of the liquid has been cooked off of the mixture.

Makes 4 servings.

NUTRITIONAL ANALYSIS PER SERVING:

Calories—83	Protein—0.8 g	Magnesium—8 mg	Omega-6—0.05 g
Total Fat—0.3 g	Iron—0.3 mg	Potassium—144 mg	Folate—7 mcg
Carbohydrates—20.9 g	Sodium—147 mg	Vitamin C—7.6 mg	
Dietary Fiber—1.3 g	Calcium—11 mg	Omega-3—0.01 g	

Plums contain the healthy compounds sorbitol and isatin. Known health benefits include regulating the functioning of the digestive system. Plums are also a source of vitamin A, beta-carotene, and phenolic antioxidants (zeaxanthin), which are essential for good eyesight and in the prevention of lung and oral cavity cancers.

ROASTED PEARS AND PARSNIPS

This unlikely pairing is a pleasant surprise of nutty and sweet, crunchy and savory. Similar to the Pears and Beets recipe, parsnips add an earthy taste to this dish. Parsnips are not common to the American diet. But don't let that deter you. They are very easy to cook. This match is sure to please.

Ingredients:

2 pears, sliced

3 parsnips, diced

Salt, pinch

2 tbs extra virgin olive oil

½ cup hazelnuts, chopped

Directions:

Toss parsnips with olive oil and salt. Place on oven sheet and roast for 20 minutes or until soft. Slice pears into eight slices and place in a mixing bowl. Combine parsnips, pear slices, hazelnuts. Mix.

Makes 4 servings.

NUTRITIONAL ANALYSIS PER SERVING:

Calories—266	Protein—4 g	Magnesium—61 mg	Omega-6—2 g
Total Fat—17.4 g	Iron—1.4 mg	Potassium—563 mg	Folate—91 mcg
Carbohydrates—27 g	Sodium—10 mg	Vitamin C—20.3 mg	
Dietary Fiber—8.7 g	Calcium—58 mg	Omega-3—0.1 g	

Parsnips are a great source of potassium and fiber. They also are a good source of vitamin C, which can help in stimulating bowel movement. In addition, this recipe provides vitamins E and K, copper, and manganese.

DESSERTS

COCOA PUDDING

This delightful dessert has all the right ingredients. Rich and creamy, it is quick to make with a light chocolate flavor and the texture of mousse. It contains a great amount of fiber and is an excellent source of good fats.

Ingredients:

½ cup walnuts

½ cup cocoa nibs

¼ tsp turmeric

1 tbs flaxseeds

1 cup of coconut milk, vanilla

½ avocado

2 to 3 dates, Medjool, pitted, sliced

2 tbs blueberries

Optional: 1 tsp of creamy peanut butter

Directions:

Add to the blender or food processor the walnuts, cocoa, nibs, turmeric, and flaxseeds. Blend until the mixture is pulverized. Add the remaining ingredients (not the peanut butter) and blend until texture is consistent. Scrape contents into a bowl and refrigerate for 1 to 2 hours.

Serve topped with peanut butter if desired.

Makes 4 servings.

NUTRITIONAL ANALYSIS PER SERVING:

Calories—184	Protein—5.3 g	Magnesium—106 mg	Omega-6—1.5 g
Total Fat—12.9 g	Iron—2.3 mg	Potassium—565 mg	Folate—40 mcg
Carbohydrates—20.8 g	Sodium—68 mg	Vitamin C—4.6 mg	
Dietary Fiber—8.5 g	Calcium—51 mg	Omega-3—4.5 g	

This recipe is an excellent source of omega-3 fatty acids making it a natural anti-inflammatory. It also contains a good amount of copper.

BAKED BANANAS WITH CINNAMON AND CHOCOLATE

Every once in a while, we would like to have a dessert. This recipe provides sweet taste while helping to control blood sugar. But do not be fooled—this dish is decadent with its dark chocolate and aromatic spices of cardamom and cinnamon. A little goes a long way.

Ingredients:

2 bananas, sliced into halves

1 tsp cardamom

1 tsp cinnamon

2 tbs coconut oil

¼ cup chocolate, dark

Directions:

Heat the oven to 375 degrees. Place banana slices on a cookie sheet. Add the coconut oil, cardamom and cinnamon to the bananas. Bake for 15 minutes. While the banana is baking, melt chocolate. Drizzle the chocolate onto the banana slices when they come out of the oven. Enjoy.

Makes 4 servings.

NUTRITIONAL ANALYSIS PER SERVING:

Calories—195	Protein—1.3 g	Magnesium—33 mg	Omega-6—0.2 g
Total Fat—7.3 g	Iron—0.7 mg	Potassium—281 mg	Folate—9 mcg
Carbohydrates—34 g	Sodium—14 mg	Vitamin C—6.3 mg	
Dietary Fiber—2.8 g	Calcium—15 mg	Omega-3—0.02 g	

The cinnamon added to this recipe is not just for flavor. Cinnamon helps regulate blood sugar levels.

ROASTED PEARS WITH WALNUTS, CINNAMON, AND DATES

You will love this roasted pear dish. The stuffing is absolutely delicious and rich, and a small bit is satisfying. I love roasting fruits and vegetables, like in this recipe—the heat brings out the natural sweetness and flavors.

Ingredients:

¼ cup walnuts, chopped

2 tbs flaxseeds, ground

¼ tsp cinnamon

½ cup fresh dates, chopped

2 pears, halved, center scooped

Optional: 1 tsp molasses

Directions:

Heat oven to 375 degrees. In a bowl, mix walnuts, flaxseeds, cinnamon, and chopped dates. On a cookie sheet, arrange the halved pears, and add a heaping tablespoon of the walnut date mixture to the scooped centers. Bake for 15 minutes. You may add the molasses at this point if you desire.

Makes 4 servings.

NUTRITIONAL ANALYSIS PER SERVING:

Calories—144	Protein—2.1 g	Magnesium—42 mg	Omega-6—2.1 g
Total Fat—4.6 g	Iron—1 mg	Potassium—305 mg	Folate—16 mcg
Carbohydrates—27.5 g	Sodium—2 mg	Vitamin C—2.6 mg	
Dietary Fiber—6.8 g	Calcium—67 mg	Omega-3—1 g	

This recipe contains a good amount of manganese.

SNACKS

SPIRULINA SMOOTHIE

Not your average green drink, this thick and rich smoothie provides an amazing amount of electrolytes and a good source of fiber. This drink is full-bodied and has an overall nutty flavor with notes of fruit.

Ingredients:

1 cup coconut water
½ cup tart cherry juice
¼ cup pumpkin seeds
½ cup blueberries
½ avocado
¼ cup hemp seeds
1 banana
1 tbs spirulina powder

Directions:

To blender add all the ingredients. Turn on high and blend until the consistency is even. Enjoy.

Makes 4 servings.

NUTRITIONAL ANALYSIS PER SERVING:

Calories—423	Protein—13.3 g	Magnesium—209 mg	Omega-6—7.8 g
Total Fat—24.6 g	Iron—3.6 mg	Potassium—1,044 mg	Folate—112 mcg
Carbohydrates—46.3 g	Sodium—173 mg	Vitamin C—15.1 mg	
Dietary Fiber—10.3 g	Calcium—73 mg	Omega-3—0.2 g	

This smoothie contains a wonderful amount of fiber, protein and potassium. In addition, the seeds and spirulina are responsible for the good omega 3 and 6 content.

COCONUT WATER SMOOTHIE

When it is hot outside or you are feeling depleted, this is a perfect pick me up. While very simple to make, this beverage is packed with nutrition and great taste. It is truly refreshing, and your body will love you for drinking it.

Ingredients:

8 ounces coconut water

1 cup of blueberries

¼ cup chia seeds

1 tbs ground flaxseeds

Optional: 1 tbs hemp seeds

Directions:

Add all ingredients to a blender. Blend for one to two minutes until even consistency results.

Makes 4 servings.

NUTRITIONAL ANALYSIS PER SERVING:

Calories—416	Protein—13.9 g	Magnesium—291 mg	Omega-6—4 g
Total Fat—22.5 g	Iron—5.8 mg	Potassium—938 mg	Folate—46 mcg
Carbohydrates—45.9 g	Sodium—251 mg	Vitamin C—13.6 mg	
Dietary Fiber—26.6 g	Calcium—443 mg	Omega-3—12.4 g	

Besides being a wonderful source of electrolytes, the recipe is also a good source of the amino acids tryptophan, methionine, and cysteine (detoxifiers and liver support), vitamin B_1, manganese, copper, and selenium.

FRUIT (WITH PROTEIN) SALAD

All the ingredients in this crispy, crunchy fruit and protein salad work well together. It is easy to make and tastes refreshing. The protein in the salad, besides adding a nutty flavor, also adds fiber that helps decrease insulin surges.

Ingredients:

½ cup blueberries, organic

½ banana, sliced

½ cup of cantaloupe, diced

¼ cup walnuts

¼ cup sunflower seeds

¼ cup Chia seeds

Mint, fresh, minced

Squeeze of lemon

Directions:

Mix all ingredients together except the lemon juice. Squeeze the lemon juice onto the surface of the fruit either in the serving bowl or in individual bowls.

Makes 4 servings.

NUTRITIONAL ANALYSIS PER SERVING:

Calories—401	Protein—10.9 g	Magnesium—183 mg	Omega-6—9.6 g
Total Fat—24.6 g	Iron—3.8 mg	Potassium—508 mg	Folate—79 mcg
Carbohydrates—40.8 g	Sodium—15 mg	Vitamin C—18.4 mg	
Dietary Fiber—14.1 g	Calcium—211 mg	Omega-3—6 g	

This recipe contains a good source of the amino acid tryptophan, and vitamins A, E, and B_1, and copper and manganese.

SPEARMINT, STRAWBERRY, AND ORANGE ICED TEA

Afternoon delight. This is a refreshing drink that will help with hydration. This tea is bright and refreshing with gentle notes of fruit.

Ingredients:

1 spearmint teabag

1 green teabag

4 slices (⅛ of inch) of an orange

4 to 6 strawberries slices

4 cups of water

Stevia or maple syrup to taste

Directions:

Boil water and then cut heat off. Add the teabags to the water in the pot. Let steep for 3 to 4 minutes, and then remove the teabags. Add orange slices and sliced strawberries and let steep for 20 to 30 minutes. Strain all solids out and place fluid into a container and refrigerate until cool or cold.

Makes 4 servings.

NUTRITIONAL ANALYSIS PER SERVING:

Calories—41	Protein—0.7 g	Magnesium—16 mg	Omega-6—0 g
Total Fat—0.1 g	Iron—0.2 mg	Potassium—222 mg	Folate—39 mcg
Carbohydrates—10.4 g	Sodium—8 mg	Vitamin C—48.4 mg	
Dietary Fiber—1.8 g	Calcium—32 mg	Omega-3—0 g	

Spearmint tea supports digestion, boosts respiratory health, and helps to relieve stress. Spearmint contains a very good level of iron—more than 100% of the daily recommended amount. Menthol is one of the active ingredients in spearmint and has a soothing and sedative effect on the body.

BROTH WITH OKRA AND BEET GREENS

This warm and soothing broth is meant to be a daily tonic that I use extensively in my practice. Its flavor is comforting and refreshing. Many patients have adopted it as their morning drink.

Ingredients:

Chicken bones, roasted (long bones opened to expose marrow)

1 bunch of parsley

1 bunch of cilantro

1 bunch of beet greens (from 4 beets)

4 carrots

1 onion

1 garlic head

1 cup of okra (fresh or frozen)

2 yellow squash, sliced and quartered

4 to 8 quarts of water

Directions:

Place bones in 4 to 8 quarts of water. Break open the long bones to expose the marrow. Place all the vegetables in the water and bone mixture, turn heat to a simmer. Simmer for 8 to 12 hours. Strain all solids from the liquid broth (save the liquid and discard the solids). Drink warm.

You may store this broth in the refrigerator up to 4 days. It stores well up to 3 months in the freezer.

Serving size: 1 cup

NUTRITIONAL ANALYSIS PER SERVING:

Calories—41

Micronutrient and electrolytes during surgery and other phases of treatment are very important to the healing process. Bone broths contain a high amount of potassium, magnesium, calcium, and other nutrients.

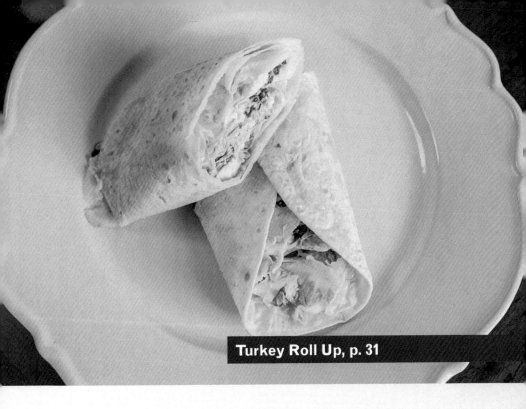
Turkey Roll Up, p. 31

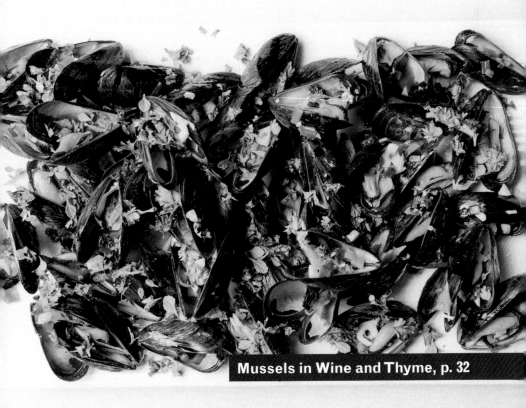
Mussels in Wine and Thyme, p. 32

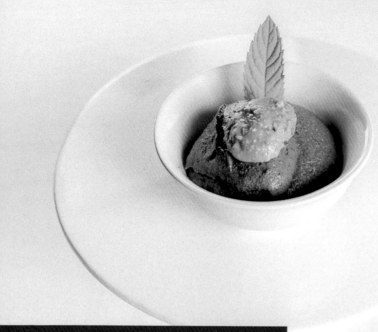

Cocoa Pudding, p. 51

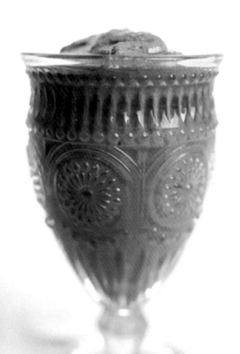

Spirulina Smoothie, p. 54

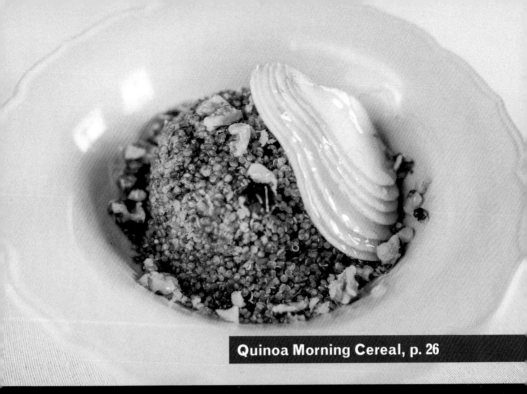

Quinoa Morning Cereal, p. 26

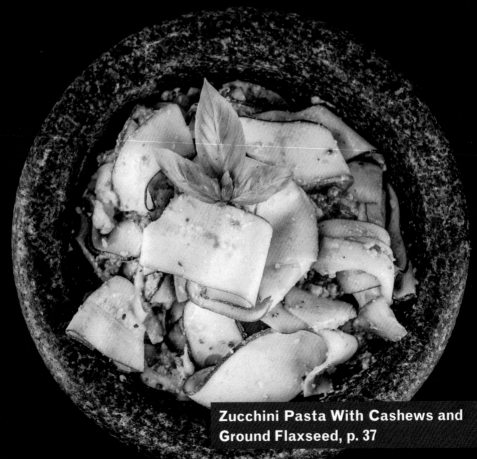

Zucchini Pasta With Cashews and
Ground Flaxseed, p. 37

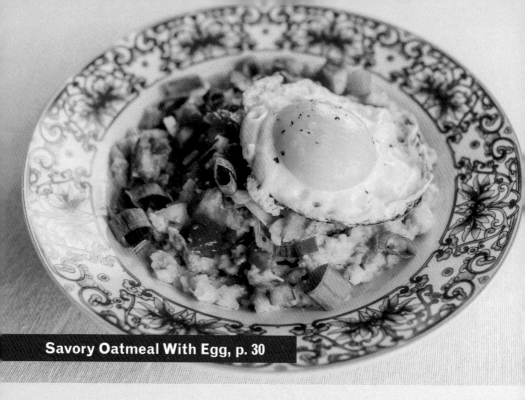

Savory Oatmeal With Egg, p. 30

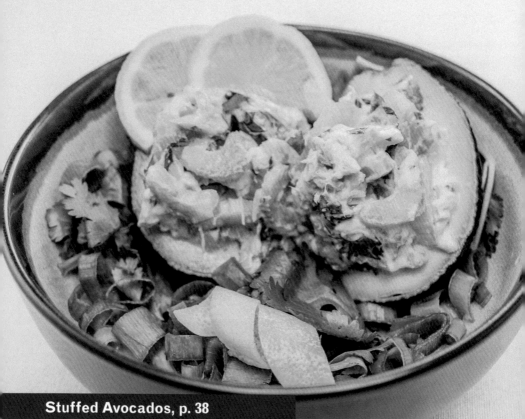

Stuffed Avocados, p. 38

CHAPTER 4

Getting Stronger: Exercise for Patients With Prostate Cancer

The first step toward change is awareness. The second step is acceptance.
—Nathaniel Brandon

A well-rounded exercise plan that includes physical activity at least 5 days a week delivers solid health benefits. Physical activity is essential not only in cancer remission, but also in addressing side effects from treatment. Prostate cancer treatment in general can result in problems with sexual function, depression, mood, weight gain, decreased muscle mass, metabolic syndrome (prediabetes), fatigue, and osteoporosis. Effects from regular exercise counters these symptoms through improving self-esteem, circulation, stabilizing mood, decreasing depression and anxiety, increasing bone strength, decreasing pain, and improving sexual function. Most important to avoid recurrence and extend remission, exercise helps to improve immune function. In summary, studies have found that regular exercise improves cancer-specific quality of life and cancer-specific fatigue.

Sexual concerns, one of the greatest sources of concern for men, include change in body image, partner relationships, sex drive, sexual performance, and masculinity. Exercise contributes to acceptance of sexual change through affirming strength-based aspects of masculinity and peer support. Furthermore, men who exercise regularly have better erectile and sexual function.

Regular exercise is particularly beneficial for men on androgen/hormone therapy for advanced prostate cancer. It addresses weight gain, diabetes development, and heart disease. Certain types of exercise, like weight bearing exercise, have also been shown to decrease bone loss.

Resistance and aerobic exercise programs can reverse muscle loss in men undergoing androgen suppression therapy for prostate cancer. Exercise also preserves physical function in prostate cancer patients with bone metastases.

Studies have definitively concluded that exercise can improve quality of life and reduce fatigue in prostate cancer patients. For example, patients undergoing radiation therapy for localized prostate cancer who participated in a cardiovascular exercise program for 8 weeks improved their cardiovascular fitness, flexibility, muscle strength, and overall quality of life. They also experienced less fatigue than patients who did not exercise.

Researchers have found that the exercise does not have to be vigorous to be beneficial. Scottish researchers determined that moderate-intensity walking produced a significant improvement in physical functioning with no significant increase in fatigue. Improved physical functioning, they wrote, may be necessary to combat the fatigue that comes with radiation therapy. Fatigue and decreased stamina associated with cancer treatment are associated with loss of muscle mass. Fatigue associated with muscle loss is also associated with increased risk of developing osteopenia and osteoporosis.

Regarding immune function, physical activity can directly affect tumor cell growth by positively affecting inflammatory responses in the tumor mass microenvironment. This is an extremely important finding as it relates to recurrence and remission.

Exercise has also been shown to affect treatment outcome and remission. A recent study by Stacey Kenfield, ScD, looked at survival after diagnoses of prostate cancer and found that men who were more active lived longer overall and had less probability of dying of prostate cancer. We know that moderate to vigorous exercise 5 to 6 days a week is important to improve quality of life and overall health and is the recommendation by the American Cancer Society.

Other studies have suggested that more physically active men may have a lower risk of prostate cancer—or prostate cancer progression—than less active or sedentary men.

The researchers looked at the impact of vigorous activity on different types of prostate cancer at various ages. They found that men ages 65 or older who engaged in at least 3 hours of vigorous physical activity a week reduced their risk of being diagnosed with high-grade, advanced, or fatal prostate cancer by nearly 70%.

The findings were consistent with an earlier study by the American Cancer Society, which followed 72,174 men for 9 years. Researchers found no difference in the overall risk of prostate cancer between men who engaged in the most physical activity and those who reported no physical activity. But when it came to aggressive prostate cancer, physical activity appeared protective: Men who got the most exercise were 31% less likely to develop aggressive disease than men who opted for the sofa. A 2006 Norwegian study yielded a similar result.

A 2005 San Francisco study took a slightly different tack in examining the exercise–cancer relationship. Rather than follow participants over time, researchers randomly assigned 93 men with low-grade prostate cancer who were pursuing active surveillance to one of two groups: a control group that received standard care and an experimental group that was asked to make comprehensive lifestyle changes, including the initiation of an exercise program. Their results suggested that exercise may slow the progression of low-grade prostate cancer.

Before we get started, let us make sure we are ready:

- You should check with your doctor before starting any exercise program. Make sure your doctor clears you for the exercise plan that you will be engaging in.

- For some exercises that are new to you, for example, weight lifting, it might be wise to consult with (and/or hire) a trainer. This will ensure you get guidance on correct techniques, which will lead to better results and less risk of injury.

- For some of the exercises you will need proper equipment. The best places for these are private or public gym facilities. The YMCA in many places has a free program for cancer patients called the Live Strong Program. A grant allows all cancer patients and survivors to enroll in a free 6-week program and use of the YMCA.

- Many of the exercises call for measuring your maximum heart rate. Here is how you find it: 220 − (your age) = Maximum heart rate.

- Before beginning any exercise, you should always include a warm up of stretching or engaging in the activity at a very low intensity. This will help to prevent injury.

- When putting together your exercise plan, you may choose to focus on just one type of exercise, or you might want to include a variety. Best results are achieved from doing some form of exercise at least five times a week 30 to 40 minutes a day on a regular and consistent basis. This should be your goal, but you should start gradually, obtaining your goal over time.

RESISTANT EXERCISE AND HIGH REPETITION WEIGHTS

Resistance exercise is a promising approach to counteract loss of muscle mass, muscle strength, and physical performance in patients suffering from prostate cancer and its treatment-related side effects. These exercises should play a large role in cancer rehabilitation and care of patients.

Studies confirm 1 year of resistance training improved muscle strength in androgen-deprived prostate cancer survivors. Findings from this study contribute to the mounting evidence that resistance exercise should become a routine part of clinical care, especially in older men with advanced prostate cancer.

What Is It?

There are several styles of resistance exercise. For our concerns, we focus on weight lifting and any other exercise that uses the body's own weight as a resistance. Resistance training is any exercise that causes the muscles to contract against an external resistance with the expectation of increases in strength, tone, mass, and/or endurance. The external resistance can be handheld weights, exercise bands, your own body weight, bricks, bottles of water, or any other object that causes the muscles to contract.

Resistance training works by causing microscopic damage or tears to the muscle cells, which in turn are quickly repaired by the body to help the muscles regenerate and grow stronger.

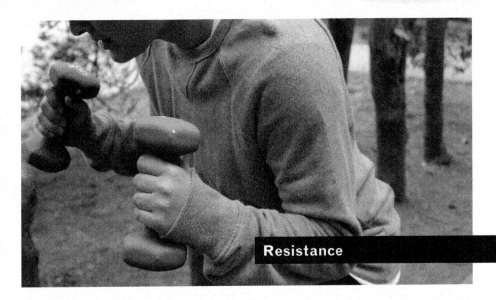

Resistance

What Is It Good For?

The American College of Sports Medicine promotes resistance training for the physical benefits of increased strength, endurance, and improved body composition. Further, self-confidence, injury reduction, performance enhancement, and reduced risk of falls are by-products of resistance training. Muscle tone and definition are common goals of resistance training exercisers. These benefits are made possible by a variety of resistance training protocols including that of high-repetition low-weight exercises.

High-resistance low-repetition programs primarily increase muscle strength and a low-resistance high-repetition program increases muscle endurance. Twelve to 15 repetitions of a light load, and eight to 10 repetitions of a moderate load per set of three are recommended by the American College of Sports Medicine. Resistance training protocols with ranges over 15 repetitions, including 20 and 30 or more repetitions per set, are utilized in research though are less prescribed for exercise programs.

A study published in April 2012 issue of the *Journal for Applied Physiology* concluded that lifting less weight for more repetitions is as effective as lifting heavier weights for lower reps. An earlier study published in the August 2010 issue of the journal *PLoS ONE* went one step further and concluded that lifting light weights for high reps is more effective than using high weights for lower reps for inducing muscle growth. High-rep, light-weight workouts offer several benefits. They are particularly helpful for new or older exercisers or people with joint issues who might be afraid or unable to lift heavier weights. Even experienced lifters can benefit from incorporating this type of training into their workouts.

Suggested Plan

This suggested plan is to get you started in resistance training. There are several exercise plans that can also help achieve the benefits. This one just helps to get you started on your journey.

Before getting started there are a few definitions to clarify. In the following, you will see an exercise plan that calls for repetitions and sets. A repetition is the number of times you will repeat an exercise over a period of time, and a confluent fashion. A set is the number of times you will repeat that number or repetitions. For example, an exercise may call for you to do 10 repetitions times four sets. This means that in the first set of the exercise you will repeat the exercise 10 times. You will likely have a short break after completing the exercise 10 times. You will go on to do another 10 repetitions. This would be your second set.

The equipment you will need for this suggested exercise plan will include: handheld weights (about 50%–60% of your maximum weight capacity), bench press, medicine ball, and a lateral pulldown machine. This is common exercise equipment found at a private gym or local YMCA.

Description of Exercises

I suggest consulting an athletic trainer if you are not familiar with any of the exercises discussed in the following. I am including a brief description, with a summary of proper technique, but it is best to check your own personal form with an expert trainer before proceeding.

Body Weight Squats—This exercise uses a person's own body weight as resistance and is done to tone and create muscle density in the legs and buttocks areas. Start by standing erect with your feet shoulder width apart. Lean slightly forward by pushing your hips back. Bend your knees slowly as you keep your back straight. Raise yourself back up when your knees are at a 70- to 90-degree angle.

Push-Ups—Push-ups help to strengthen your upper body. Start by laying on your abdomen on a hard, flat surface. Tuck your toes under and place your hands next to your chest. Tighten your abdominal muscles and push up until your arms are straight. Lower yourself and repeat.

Hand Weights—Hand weights can affect many small and large muscle groups in the upper body. You may be seated or in a standing position. It is always important to have good posture: straight back, tight abdomen. Hold hand weights securely. Raise the weights slowly until you reach the given position and lower slowly.

Plank—Planks are a great way to condition your abdominal muscles. Strong abdominal muscles help to avoid back injuries among other things. Start by laying on your abdomen on a hard surface. Tuck your toes under, and place your forearms directly beneath your shoulders, close to your body. Put your weight on your forearms and raise your body, keeping your body straight while squeezing your abdomen and buttocks. Stay as long as you can.

Bench Press—Bench presses help to develop the upper body muscles and are done with a bench and weights. You might want to initially work with a spotter, someone who can help manage the weight that will be directly over your chest. Lie on your back on the bench. Unrack the bar by straightening your arms. Lower the bar to your mid chest and press the bar up until your arms are straight.

Sit Ups—This exercise is helpful for abdominal muscles. Lay down on your back and bend your knees at a 90-degree angle. Place your hands, with bent arms, behind your ears. Tighten your abdomen and sit up in a slow steady fashion. Lower yourself slowly.

Lateral Pull Downs—Lateral pull downs are helpful for conditioning the upper body, especially the arms and back muscles. Sit down on the seat with a straight back, abdomen tight with your feet on the floor. The lateral bar should be at a height so that your outstretched arms can comfortably grasp the bar without having to fully stand up. Grasp bar with a wide grip and pull down. Squeeze your shoulder blades together. Slowly let the bar down to return to the originally position.

BEGINNER

- *Monday and Wednesday:*
- Body weight squats for 30 to 60 seconds (do as many as you can within this period of time), repeat to complete three to four sets.
- Push-ups for 30 to 60 seconds, three to four sets
- Dumb bells/hand weights bicep curls for 30 to 60 seconds, four to five sets (50%–60% of maximum weight capacity)
- Dumb bells/tricep swings for 30 to 60 seconds, four to five sets
- Plank for 20 to 40 seconds, three to four sets

INTERMEDIATE

(Once the series of Beginner exercises has become easy, add the Tuesday and Thursday routine.)

- *Tuesday and Thursday:*
- Bench presses for eight reps, three to four sets
- Sit ups/abdominal crunches for 20 reps, three sets
- Jumping jacks for 45 seconds, three sets
- Lateral Pulldown for 10 reps, three sets

FAST WALKING

There are many reasons to engage in brisk walking. It quickens your heart beat, circulating more blood and oxygen to your muscles and your organs, including the brain. Experts suggest that brisk walking for 30 minutes at a moderate speed can help you burn 150 to 200 calories, not to mention that aerobic exercises like brisk walking are the major factor correlated with cancer prevention and remission!

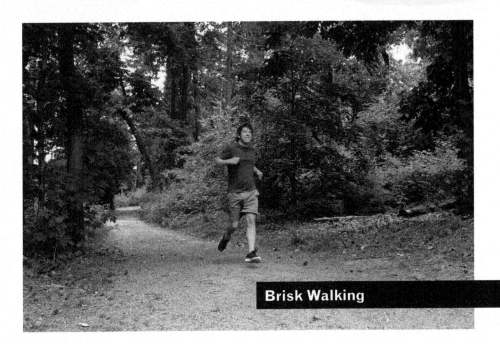

Brisk Walking

In a study of more than 1,400 men diagnosed with early stage prostate cancer, men who walked briskly (not leisurely) for at least 3 hours a week were 57% less likely to have their cancer progress than those who walked less often and less vigorously. In an analysis from the Health Professionals Follow-up Study, men diagnosed with localized prostate cancer who engaged in vigorous activity at least 3 hours each week had a 61% lower chance of dying from the illness compared to men who engaged in vigorous activity less than 1 hour a week.

According to a study by the Harvard Medical School, walking for just 2.5 hours a week, which is 21 minutes a day, can cut the risk of heart disease by 30%. A 2009 issue of *Harvard Men's Health Watch* reported that walking is seriously underrated. Two scientists sifted through 4,295 articles published between 1997 and 2007 on walking. Each of these studies collected information about the participants' walking habits and cardiovascular risk factors, such as age, smoking, and alcohol use. The participants were followed for 11.3 years and during this time their cardiovascular events and deaths were recorded. When scientists compiled these data, they found that walking reduced the risk of cardiovascular events by 31% and cut the risk of an early death by 32%.

Exercise is good for the brain but walking specifically is good for boosting your memory. A 2011 study published in *The Proceedings of the National Academy of Sciences* showed how walking for 40 minutes at a stretch three times a week could increase the volume of the hippocampus by 2%, which is significant. This is of interest for men experiencing brain fog associated with androgen-blocking treatments or chemotherapy.

Another study presented at the 2014 annual meeting of the American Association for the Advancement of Science found that regular brisk walks can slow down the deterioration of the brain and the faltering mental skills that old age often brings. The study was done with men and women between the ages of 60 and 80 and it concluded that taking a short walk three times a week increased the size of that part of the brain linked to planning and memory.

According to a study done at Appalachian State University in North Carolina, a moderately paced walk for about 30 to 45 minutes daily can increase the number of immune system cells in your body and, over a period of time, can have remarkable effect on your body's ability to fight disease, including cancer. To be more specific, walking at least 20 minutes a day could reduce the risk of getting sicker by almost 43%.

Researchers at the University of Colorado found that regular walking helped to prevent peripheral artery disease (which impairs blood flow in the legs and causes leg pain in one fifth of elderly people). Because walking is a weight-bearing exercise, it can also help prevent the bone disease osteoporosis, a side effect of prostate cancer treatment. Even if a 20-minute power walk at lunchtime is all you manage, after 6 weeks benefits can be seen.

Types of Walking

Nordic Walking—Nordic walking uses ski-like poles which forces people to pick up their pace and work harder, thus burning more calories and increasing muscle mass, especially in the upper body. On average, people use 20% more calories when they use poles.

Mall Walking—This was originally devised/advised by doctors, who encouraged cardiac patients to incorporate indoor walking in shopping malls to hasten their rehab. Many malls are open during the early hours of the morning prior to shop openings and during the winter months to accommodate people walking.

Treadmills—Treadmills are more well controlled and are easier on your joints than cement (running outdoors). The incline and the program can be changed for varying physical condition and injuries.

Water Walking—For patients with joint issues, water walking is an excellent option. Water walking can be safely done at a community or private pool during lane swimming hours. This type of walking is very aerobic and increases muscle mass with little impact on joints. Some people like to use a waist flotation device for added safety.

Exercise Plan

Make sure you have good walking shoes or sneakers with good tread before you begin. You may also want to wear a good pair of socks to prevent rubbing and blistering. If it is a sunny day, do not forget your sunscreen and sun hat. If you get bored easily or are a time checker, you might want to consider finding an interesting podcast or a great music playlist that lasts for the time you have allocated to walk. If you are just starting out, be cautious about over-doing it. Pace yourself.

When using walking as one of your primary exercises, there are some techniques that will help to achieve good results. Posture and breath during walking is important.

Regarding proper posture, stand tall with your arms by your sides and pull your belly in toward your spine so that your core muscles are working. Shoulders should be comfortably pulled back as opposed to caved in. Your eyes should be focused 10 to 30 feet ahead. Keep your shoulders relaxed. Bend your elbows at a 90-degree angle and cup your hands lightly, rather than clenching your fists. You should be consciously breathing in and out rather than holding your breath at any point.

Leading with the heel, step forward with your right foot and move your arms in opposition (i.e., as your left arm moves forward, your right moves back). Transfer your weight all the way through the heel of your right foot.

When you first begin your walking routine, do it on flat terrain. After a few weeks, add some hills (going up and down as well). Varying your route will also help to decrease boredom but also will work different muscles, and thus make your exercise more effective.

BEGINNER

- *Monday to Saturday:* Walk 10 minutes at a moderate pace.
- *Sunday:* Walk slowly for 20 minutes.

INTERMEDIATE

- *Monday:* Rest.
- *Tuesday to Friday:* Walk for 25 minutes at a moderate pace one day, 30 minutes the next.
- *Saturday:* Walk 20 minutes fast.
- *Sunday:* Walk 45 minutes at a moderate pace.

ADVANCED

- *Monday:* Rest.
- *Tuesday to Friday:* Walk 45 minutes at a moderate pace one day and 50 minutes the next day.
- *Saturday:* Walk 50 minutes at a fast pace.
- *Sunday:* Walk 60 minutes at a moderate pace.

Plan for Water Walking

BEGINNER

- *Monday:* Lane walk for 10 to 15 minutes at a comfortable rate.
- *Wednesday:* Lane walk for 10 to 15 minutes at a comfortable rate.

INTERMEDIATE

- *Monday:* Lane walk for 20 to 25 minutes at a brisk pace.
- *Wednesday:* Lane walk for 20 to 25 minutes at a brisk pace.
- *Friday:* Lane walk for 20 to 25 minutes at a brisk pace.

ADVANCED

- *Monday:* Lane walk for 30 to 40 minutes at a brisk pace.
- *Wednesday:* Lane walk for 30 to 40 minutes at a brisk pace.
- *Friday:* Lane walk for 30 to 40 minutes at a brisk pace.

BICYCLING

Cycling is mainly an aerobic activity, which means that your heart, blood vessels, and lungs all get a workout. You will breathe deeper, perspire, and experience increased body temperature, which will improve your overall fitness level.

There are several reasons to choose cycling as part of your exercise plan. It is low impact and thus is associated with less strain and injuries

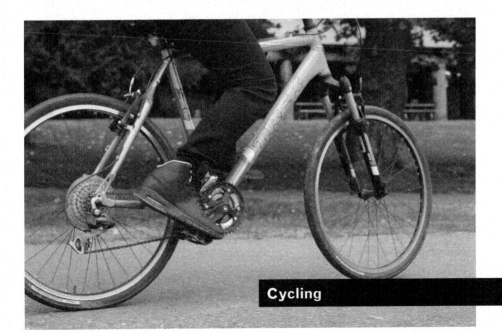

Cycling

than most other forms of exercise. It is an excellent muscle workout especially for your lower body and does not require a high level of physical skill. You can moderate the level of intensity easily and it is a very fun way to get fit. Cycling can be incorporated conveniently into your daily activities, including using it as a way of getting to work or to a store.

Why Is It Good?

The health benefits of cycling are multiple:

- Increased cardiovascular fitness
- Increased muscle strength and flexibility
- Decreased stress levels
- Strengthened bones
- Decreased body fat levels
- Increased immune function
- Reduced anxiety and depression

Cycling strengthens your heart muscles, lowers resting pulse, and reduces blood fat levels. Type 2 diabetes is a concern for men being treated over a long period for prostate cancer. Large-scale research in Finland found that people who cycled for more than 30 minutes per day had a 40% lower risk of developing diabetes.

Mental health conditions such as depression, stress, and anxiety can be reduced by regular bike riding. This is because of the exercise itself and because of the enjoyment that riding a bike can bring.

Increasing your workouts from 30 to 60 minutes is ideal. According to *Harvard Health*, a 155-pound person will burn about 520 calories per hour of bicycling at a moderate pace. The stationary bike is not the most effective cardio activity to burn calories, so longer workouts are more ideal.

There is a noted association between prostate cancer and intense cycling for 8 hours or more per week. Researchers have found that cycling less than 3.75 hours per week does not have this association and in fact have positive and beneficial biochemical changes that occur after exercise that reduce the risk of cancer.

Plan

Before you get started:

Make sure your bicycle is working properly prior to getting started. Have the brakes, the gears, and tire pressure checked. Make sure your seat is at the proper height. Your legs should not be fully extended when you are seated and your feet are in the pedals. Always wear a properly fitting helmet.

A long ride on a narrow bicycle seat compresses the nerves in the perineum, the area between the scrotum and the anus, leading to numbness in the penis. You should pick a wide seat with plenty of padding. You can also try gel-filled and anatomy-friendly seats. Some bikers also will invest in padded bike shorts to help with this issue.

Suggested Cycling Plan

Warm up by stretching for 5 to 10 minutes. Begin your bike ride with mild intensity for 5 to 10 minutes.

BEGINNER

Cycle 20 minutes on flat/no incline at 50% to 60% of maximum heart rate two to three times a week

INTERMEDIATE

Cycle 30 minutes on variable terrain with at least one hill at 60% maximum heart rate three to four times a week

ADVANCED

Cycle 40 to 60 minutes on variable terrain with at least two hills at 60% maximum heart rate three to four times a week

SWIMMING

Swimming builds endurance, muscle strength, and cardiovascular fitness, and helps maintain a healthy weight, healthy heart and lungs, tones muscles, and builds strength. It provides an all-over body workout, as nearly all of your muscles are used during swimming. Swimming requires you to reach, stretch, twist, and pull your way through the water.

Swimming is a great aerobic workout that has low impact on joints, and it can be done by both the very old and the very young. It is utilized by athletes to stay strong and keep fit when recovering from injury, and there is no fancy equipment needed.

According to the scientists, swimming can improve immunity, promote prostate local blood and lymphatic circulation, and encourage more vigorous secretion of prostatic fluid, thus contributing to lessened prostate inflammation.

For years, researchers scoffed at the idea that swimming affected bone mass. Research published in the *Journal of Applied Physiology* showed that swimming can increase or stabilize bone mass. Because there are ethical reasons to avoid in-depth bone examination on humans, the study put rats into three groups: running, swimming, and a control group with no exercise stimulation. While running still showed the highest increase in bone mineral density, the swimming group also showed benefits over the control group in both bone mineral density and femoral bone weight. While more studies are needed, these new findings show that previous research dismissing the bone benefits of swimming may need to be revisited.

Plan

I recommend that you know how to swim or take lessons before incorporating swimming as one of your main ways to work out. You will need to find a private or public swimming pool and look at the schedule for lane swimming. I recommend facilities that have an on-duty lifeguard as well.

You should plan on your goal of swimming for 30 minutes so that your actual exercise time (as opposed to rest time) ends up around 20 minutes. To begin, commit yourself to three times a week, 30 minutes per workout.

CHAPTER 5

Finding Emotional Balance: Mind–Body Therapies for Patients With Prostate Cancer

Change your thoughts and you change your world.

—Norman Vincent Peale

I felt absolutely lost when I got my diagnosis. I frankly was in denial. I had just started a new relationship and didn't want to lose that because of changes in sexual function or because of some of the side effects I heard about. I kept putting off treatment until my sister talked me into going to see a mental health counselor. He helped me to work through my fears and make a plan. The plan helped me feel like I had some control of the diagnosis. I started treatment shortly after that. I'm doing currently doing well, and I still have my relationship.

—T. S.

The diagnosis of prostate cancer can deeply affect men's emotional well-being and can lead to depression and anxiety. Men are often worried about changes to sexual health, and emasculation, and therefore their relationships. They may even feel guilt and loss of identity relative to their partners or spouses. Psychological distress can also result from uncertainty of the course of the disease, fearing progression or recurrence. Luckily, there are some ways to help men regain a sense of balance and control.

Mind–body therapies can affect quality of life by reducing stress and empowering patients. This leads to patients who are better able to manage their lives, moods, relationships, and overall well-being.

For some men, the use of mind–body therapies is foreign and uncomfortable, and as a result they might be very resistant to using them. However, these therapies have been shown through research and through observation to be instrumental in helping men restore some normalcy to their lives and improve sexual intimacy and self-esteem after a cancer diagnosis.

In general, the objective of using mind–body therapies for prostate cancer patients is to decrease stress, increase reproductive function, increase libido, increase immune function.

Several different types of mind–body therapies will be summarized with general frequency recommendations. Because these therapies are complex, you should find classes, teachers, or videos that can explain or demonstrate more in depth.

YOGA

Yoga does not require fancy clothing or the ability to bend your leg behind your head to get started. To the contrary in traditional practices, yoga is noncompetitive, focusing on nonjudgment and starting where you are.

According to the National Center for Complementary and Integrative Health, around 91% of American adults—21 million—used yoga in 2012. A clinical trial study suggests that doing yoga twice a week may improve quality of life for men being treated for prostate cancer and can help reduce the side effects of radiation, which includes fatigue, sexual dysfunction, and urinary incontinence. Yoga improves the pelvic floor muscles and increases circulation. Decades of research show that yoga can reduce the emotional and physical fatigue brought on by cancer treatment. Now, researchers have shown for the first time that is also true specifically for men being treated for prostate cancer. Men who took a yoga class twice a week during treatment reported less fatigue, fewer sexual side effects, and better urinary functioning than men who did not. "The data are convincing," said the study's principal investigator, Dr. Neha Vapiwala, an associate professor of radiation oncology at the University of Pennsylvania School of Medicine in Philadelphia.

"What we need now is a better understanding of how and why yoga produces these benefits."

Vapiwala and her colleagues enrolled 50 men with early or advanced nonmetastatic prostate cancer who ranged in age from 53 to 85. Among them, 22 were assigned to the yoga group and the rest were not. All the men got scheduled radiation treatments during the study, 29 were also on hormonal therapy, and 19 had previously been treated surgically for prostate cancer. The groups were evenly balanced with respect to cancer treatments, in addition to other possible treatments for erectile and urinary problems. Men who already practiced yoga or were treated previously with radiation were ineligible for the study, as were men with metastatic prostate cancer.

Yoga is a mind–body practice with historical origins in ancient Indian philosophy. It combines physical postures, breathing techniques, and meditation or relaxation. There are many styles of yoga. A person's fitness level and desired practice outcome determines the type of yoga class for which they are best suited. Studies suggest that yoga is a safe and effective way to increase physical activity and enhance strength, flexibility, and balance. Yoga practice has also shown benefit in specific medical conditions.

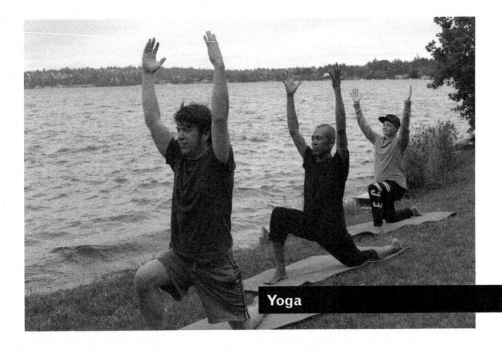

Yoga

A study investigating yoga for depression examined data, including 619 participants. The researchers concluded that yoga could be considered an effective treatment option for patients with depression.

Fatigue is one of the most frequent side effects reported by survivors of cancer and often has significant long-term consequences. Research indicates that yoga can produce invigorating effects on physical and mental energy, and thereby may improve fatigue.

Yoga has been shown to reduce inflammation and may help improve symptoms of urinary urgency. More research is necessary to demonstrate the effectiveness of yoga to reduce urinary incontinence symptoms.

Elevated levels of cortisol, the stress hormone related to depressing immune function, are commonly seen in depression, and yoga has demonstrated an ability to decrease cortisol and stress.

There are many types of yoga. I would recommend that if you have never done yoga before or if you are recovering from cancer treatment that you try Hatha yoga. It is more simple, great for beginners, and can be easily individualized.

Look for studios in your area that offer Hatha yoga. Find a teacher and a class in which you feel welcome and comfortable. Many classes and teachers are trained in poses and accommodations for cancer patients.

To begin with, you should try to incorporate yoga into your weekly regimen twice a week and work up to at least three times or more per week.

Resources

https://www.yogaalliance.org
https://www.youtube.com/watch?v=iY4CJK40kN0
https://www.youtube.com/watch?v=V1hbqmbw1xA

GUIDED MEDITATION

Meditation can be defined as a practice of focusing one's mind to achieve mental clarity and emotional calm. It helps you to concentrate on the present moment rather than the past or the future. Meditation is seen by many researchers as potentially one of the most effective forms of stress reduction. It has been shown to affect quality of life, immune function, and improvement in mental health.

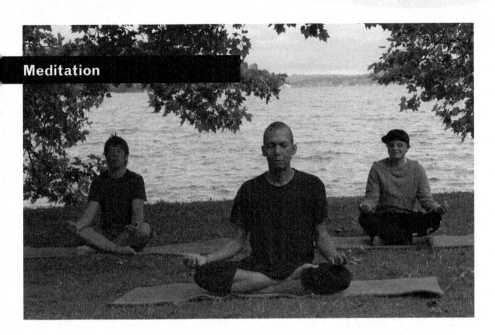

Meditation

Meditation is often referred to as a practice because to obtain that concentration is easier said than done, but with time can be obtained. Sometimes meditation is called "sitting," because one sits in a quiet location over a period, usually 10 to 20 minutes, clearing the mind. For many beginners, the most difficult part of the practice is to get their minds to be still, free of chatter. This is also the reason many are noncompliant. Because of this, I recommend guided meditation.

Guided meditation involves a trained guide or teacher either in person or as a sound recording, video, or other audio–video media. It is one of the easiest ways to enter into a state of deep relaxation and inner stillness because your own chatter is displaced by the guide's voice. I often recommend guided meditation for people having sleep disturbances as well.

I recommend using guided meditation once to twice a day, in the morning after waking and in the evening right before bed. Listed here are some of my favorite resources.

Resources

http://marc.ucla.edu/mindful-meditations
https://www.tarabrach.com/guided-meditations/
https://chopra.com/meditation

COUNSELING

Therapy, also called psychotherapy or counseling, is the process of meeting with a mental health professional to resolve or become equipped with tools to address problematic behavior, fear, beliefs, feelings, relationship problems, and more. A mental health professional can greatly help a patient cope with the emotional impact of a cancer diagnosis and the changes associated with treatment on men's and their families' lives. Counselors can help patients find words to articulate their emotions and become better equipped to manage their treatment decisions and physical changes and come to terms with them. Counseling can be one-on-one, family counseling, or a group support setting.

There are professionals specifically trained to work with cancer patients. For example, oncology social workers can provide counseling that addresses education and expected emotional outcomes. However, a professional mental health counselor can also adequately help you.

Specifically, studies have shown that counseling programs and therapy improved the sex lives of prostate cancer patients and survivors. Some studies also showed significant improvement in both partner's sexual function.

What you can expect in a counseling session is that you will be listened to, but more importantly, that your therapist will help you understand where your anxiety, grief, sadness, or whatever emotion is originating. They will establish goals to address these emotions and determine steps on how to get there. All therapy is confidential. Most mental health professionals will recommend consistent, ongoing sessions, but that all depends on the patient's needs.

When searching for a professional mental health therapist, make sure the therapist is a good match for you. Meet with the therapist before scheduling an actual appointment. Often a bad match can ruin a counseling experience for a new patient and deter men from ever using this therapy again.

Resources

https://www.counseling.org/
http://www.amhca.org/home

TAI CHI

Tai chi comes from China and is a form of exercise that involves a series of movements performed in a slow, focused manner involving deep breathing and meditation. Also known as moving meditation, tai chi was originally developed as a form of self-defense.

Each of the movements flows into the next. Movements are usually circular with relaxed muscles and slightly bent joints. A tai chi class might include easy motions, such as shoulder circles, turning the head from side to side, or rocking back and forth, help you to loosen your muscles and joints and focus on your breath and body, and sets of movements that may include a dozen or fewer movements or longer forms that may include hundreds. Different styles require smaller or larger movements. A short form with smaller, slower movements is usually recommended at the beginning, especially if you are older or not in good condition.

Benefits

- Balance is improved because of increased upper and lower body muscular strength and endurance. Flexibility, particularly in older adults, is improved, thus preventing falls.
- Investigators have found that individuals who practiced tai chi regularly had a higher aerobic capacity.
- Stress relief comes from the breathing, movement, and mental concentration, all of which help with mind–body connect ions that improve and promote calmness.
- Improved joint health.

Specifically, prostate cancer research shows that tai chi can have a positive affect on lower urinary tract symptoms, quality of life, testosterone levels, immune function, anxiety, and pain in cancer patients and survivors.

Resources

http://www.americantaichi.org/about.asp
https://www.smartaichi.com/worldtaichiday/Associations.html
https://www.youtube.com/watch?v=9Q5GYpRKNm8
https://www.youtube.com/watc<C>h?v=T0QLTOo80fE&t=32s

QI GONG

Qi gong is a breath-focused gentle exercise combined with meditation; it was developed a very long time ago in China. There are three main elements of qi gong exercise:

- Slow fluid movements that mimic movements in nature. These exercises stretch and strengthen.
- Deep breathing
- A meditative state of mind

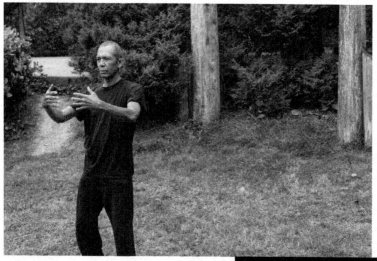

Qi Gong

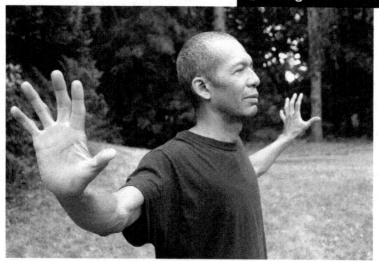

Qi gong most recently has been found to have a significant affect on prostate cancer patients and improving fatigue associated with treatment. A small study at the Huntsman Cancer Institute at the University of Utah confirmed benefits of qi gong on prostate cancer. Participants practiced qi gong two times a week for 60 minutes per session. Other positive effects include mood, pain management, decreased inflammation, and improved cognitive function.

Resources

https://www.nqa.org/
https://www.qigonginstitute.org/
https://www.youtube.com/watch?v=KcdcqW27RUs

CHAPTER 6

Seeking Resiliency and Balance: Tying It All Together

Persistence and resiliency only come from having been given the chance to work through difficult problems.

—*Gever Tulley*

This book presented a holistic and complementary plan for men who have been diagnosed with prostate cancer and who are in conventional treatment, including the watch-and-wait option. It intended to provide a variety of safe and researched therapies that help decrease or prevent side effects associated with treatment and address emotional well-being. In addition, some suggestions are also meant to be incorporated over a lifetime for decreased risk of occurrence and to maximize quality of life.

I have been able to supply you with quite a bit of information in a relatively small amount of space. Be cautious about thinking that you must incorporate everything at once. That is not how lifelong habits are formed and successful compliance achieved. Small consistent steps and a little self-understanding go a long way, especially if these things are new to you.

For example, one of my patients, whom I will call Larry, initially came to see me after having been diagnosed with prostate cancer and with prodding from his significant other. He came in a state of discourage-ment and hopelessness, wondering if there were anything that he could do to stop the progression or growth of the cancer. He was terrified that androgen hormone therapy would wreck his quality of life. He was in a state of depression.

Prior to the cancer diagnosis, Larry lived life in the fast lane. He drove and traveled a lot for work, got very little exercise, and many of his meals were on the run and from restaurants. His stress level was high, and the amount of sleep he got was well under the amount needed. His fluid intake consisted mostly of coffee with some consistent social drinking weekly. Larry was relatively young and had never been diagnosed with any other chronic health condition.

Not only was Larry in shock, but he also did not have the tools or guidance to assist him with the fall out of a cancer diagnosis and treatment.

Once Larry understood the effects his treatment was having on him, and that there were ways to reduce or prevent those side effects, he was more motivated to make changes. We started small and focused on adding consistent exercise that he enjoyed, along with having him increase his sleep.

His family helped, committing to making and eating dinner at home as a family at least three times a week. Not only was this a change to more wholesome meals, but it was a way to connect with family and foster support and togetherness as opposed to isolation in his disease. Small dietary changes continued to occur, and later in the process, as Larry saw that plant-based meals could be tasty and flavorful, he began to participate in making even more healthy changes to his diet.

Larry's dietary and exercise changes were effective in reducing many symptoms; however, his depression and anxiety still persisted. Not as much as they had to begin with, but nonetheless, enough that they affected his quality of life. Mind–body therapies were the hardest for Larry to consider using. They were new to him and there was a stigma associated with them for Larry.

It was a fellow patient that convinced Larry to try a support group of other prostate cancer patients. He attended his first support group and continued returning monthly. Months later, he suggested to his wife that they go see a counselor specially trained to work with prostate cancer patients and their spouses.

As Larry moved through counseling, his high anxiety and depression began to lift. He developed a deeper sense of self and an acceptance of changes that had occurred.

Most importantly, from all the holistic therapies that Larry employed—dietary, exercise, and mind–body solutions, he developed greater resiliency and balance in his life. He was able to turn from despair to solutions—something I wish for all prostate cancer patients and readers of this book.

APPENDIX

CANCER SUPPORT ORGANIZATIONS

Cancer organizations that can supply information on specific cancers and provide support during cancer treatment and beyond:

https://www.cancercare.org/support_groups/126-prostate_cancer_patient_support_group

https://www.cancer.com/prostate-cancer

http://www.ustoo.org/

https://pcainternational.org/

http://www.prostatehealthed.org/

COUNSELING AND THERAPY ASSOCIATIONS

https://www.counseling.org/

https://ahha.org/

https://www.hypnosisalliance.com/iact/

EXERCISE ASSOCIATIONS AND INSTITUTIONS

Associations devoted to physical therapies, exercise, and other activities discussed in the book that are particularly helpful after cancer treatment:

https://www.internationalyogafederation.net/fiyorganizations.html

http://www.yogahealthfoundation.org/

https://www.nqa.org/

https://www.qigonginstitute.org/category/81/national-qigong-association

http://www.americantaichi.org/about.asp

http://www.taichifoundation.org/

http://americanmeditationsociety.org/

http://www.meditationinstructors.com/

INDEX